Healing with the Seven Principles of Mindfulness:

How to Thrive and Succeed in a Complex Cancer System

By Jerome Freedman, Ph. D.

Cover drawing inspired by a photograph by Chan Phap Vu, a Scottish-American monk in the Plum Village Tradition of Zen Master Thich Nhat Hanh. The photograph was taken in Loch Muick, Scotland.

Disclaimer:

This material is copyright(c) 1997 - 2015, by Dr. Jerome Freedman, Ph. D. All Rights Reserved. This document is meant to be a description of the author's experience and he in no way takes responsibility for the accuracy or completeness of any medical knowledge. The author assumes no responsibility for choices made by any of the readers of this material.

The author is not a physician and makes no claims about the potential usefulness of the subject matter herein to have any medical benefit. Please check with your doctor if you find something interesting that you would like to try.

His primary purpose is to introduce you to the possibility of becoming your own advocate for medical care by adopting the *Seven Principles of Mindfulness in Healing*.

TABLE OF CONTENTS

FOREWORD BY DR. MARTIN ROSSMAN, MD

Jerome Freedman has been a friend of mine for about 30 years. His beloved son, Micah, is about to get married in his late 40's, after surviving a Stage 4 cancer at the age of seven. His miraculous recovery was not likely due to his medical treatment, and he was featured on a TV show at the time because it was so rare. Besides overseeing his medical care, Jerome brought in alternative therapies and healers and led Micah through what he calls "mind stories" (guided imagery) every day.

Jerome himself was diagnosed with bladder cancer (cancer runs strongly in his family) 18 years ago when the standard treatment was removing the bladder. He found a Harvard professor (Dr. William U. Shipley) who was researching a new "bladder-sparing" treatment got him to agree to supervise his treatment with Jerome's local Urologist, who had never done this before. Jerome still has his bladder, and, at nearly 76 years old, his good health. In the course of his recovery he has utilized every one of the Seven Principles of Healing that he teaches in this book.

Jerome is not a medical doctor, but a doctor of computer science – he's a very smart man. He's also an ordained practitioner in a Buddhist tradition and a compassionate listener and observer of the human condition. He has helped many friends and acquaintances navigate their way through cancer diagnosis, treatment, and often, recovery.

As a physician who has practiced holistic medicine, now called Integrative Medicine, for over 4 decades, I can attest to the value of the principles that Dr. Freedman recommends including in your treatment program. Some of the principles will be critical to some while others will be more important for others, but they all merit serious consideration. They all can have potentially important roles to play in your survival.

I think of an Integrative approach to cancer care this way – conventional medicine is largely aimed at eliminating cancer cells, usually through surgery, radiation, or chemotherapy, and the rest of these seven principles are aimed at supporting the healing ability of the patient who has the cancer. Whether through nutrition, alternative medicines, mind/body medicine, social support or the creation of meaning, each of these options have the potential to increase your vitality, immune responsiveness, and will to live.

It would be a mistake with many serious cancers to skip conventional treatments, although for some cancers, unfortunately, they have little to offer. Because these powerful treatments can have serious and significant side effects, they require a hard, discriminating assessment of the evidence of their effectiveness, and often more than one oncological opinion.

The other six principles also deserve serious consideration, but they don't require the same level of evidence of effectiveness, because they are much safer, and most of them involve little to no risk at all. Good nutrition, mind/body practices, social support, having a purpose and giving back, and utilizing natural therapies all may have an upside, and they have little downside. Most of them actually have positive side effects.

When I only practiced conventional medicine, I remember seeing cancer patients going through chemotherapy and radiation therapy. They would always look green and gaunt. Now, it's very rare to see someone look like that if they have added good mind/body/spirit healing support to their treatment program. Cancer patients I see now usually look pink and pretty healthy most of the time. Because they are better nourished, have fewer side effects, and have more support, they are more frequently able to tolerate the full recommended course of medical treatments. That in itself gives them a greater chance of surviving, and even thriving after cancer.

In my mind, "Cancer Treatment 101" consists of getting the very best medical and surgical treatments if they show benefit, and complementing that treatment with the very best health supportive treatments. So you're not only killing the cancer, you are enhancing the person's inborn healing abilities. If we think of the body as a garden, you are not only killing the bugs that are nibbling on your plants, you are also fertilizing the soil, watering regularly, eliminating deadwood, and making sure the plants get everything they need in order to thrive. I think that's what Dr. Freedman is telling you, too.

My last comment is that different things will help different people. Consider and try everything, and, in the end, concentrate on what's actually healing for YOU. While many people benefit from support groups, others find them difficult and depressing. Vegetarianism may be a healing diet for some people, but not all, and at certain times, even a vegetarian may need some of the nutrients in fish, or even red meat. A blend of physical activity and rest is usually very helpful, and the balance may be quite different for each individual in a group. Religion and spirituality are very important to many people, and are not of interest to others. If nothing else, a cancer diagnosis gives you a lot of motivation and opportunity to get to know what's actually true for you.

I had a friend and patient who had a rare and difficult to treat blood cancer many years ago. When he consulted me, he told me, "I don't want to meditate or sit around imagining myself healing. I hate sitting still and it's boring – it doesn't do anything for me except frustrate me." I said, "What does healing feel to you, then?" and he instantly said "Swimming. When I'm swimming I feel whole, and strong, and relaxed – like everything is working together." I told him that is what he should be doing, then, along with whatever other activities felt genuinely healing for HIM.

He lived 23 more years, and did not die of his cancer. I can't really say it was the swimming, because he had lots of both conventional and alternative treatments, but he told me many times over those years how important it had been for him to spend his time doing things that were healing for him. It had turned much of his life into an experience of learning what was nourishing, supportive and genuinely good for him, which was completely opposite of the dutiful life he had lived up to that point. "It's like night and day. In a funny way, cancer has taught me a lot. I wouldn't want to go through it again, nor would I wish it someone else, but it's helped me learn about what's healing for me more than anything I've ever experienced."

May you find what is healing for you.

Martin L. Rossman, MD
Mill Valley, CA
9/20/15

PROLOG

I HAVE SURVIVED

I have survived being the eldest of six children in a conservative Jewish family in St. Louis, where my mother spent her time at the synagogue and my father spent his time painting in the basement.

I have survived the bullies of the neighborhood, school and summer camp.

I have survived three left arm breaks before the age of ten and multiple childhood illness.

I have survived a lonely childhood with few friends and extreme longing to be liked, especially by pretty girls.

I have survived the death of my beloved sister at the age of 27, parents, grandparents and many others, mostly from cancer.

I have survived failing one semester of the fifth grade because I did not want to pay attention in school.

I have survived many years of Sunday school and Hebrew school and my Bar Mitzvah at the age of 13.

I have survived 4½ years of high school with zero girlfriends.

I have survived four years of undergraduate education in chemical engineering and six years of graduate education in physics.

I have survived the humiliation of having the fifth highest grade out of twenty-five candidates on a Ph. D. qualifying exams and then being asked to leave the school.

I have survived utterly failing oral exams over course work by not remembering a single thing when I was being quizzed.

I have survived a five year marriage with my son's mother.

I have survived my son's metastatic cancer of the kidney (Wilm's tumor) at the age of seven.

I have survived almost 19 years of living with bladder cancer.

I HAVE THRIVED

I have thrived on the thirty-six years of living with my wife, Mala.

I have thrived on raising my son and two daughters and watching them grow up and graduate from university.

I have thrived on meditation practices, creative visualization, and many years of tennis.

I have thrived on spending two summers with Father Eli in the Ozark Mountains where I learned to train people how to enter a deep state of relaxation and do creative visualization.

I have thrived on spending four months in India with Rajneesh.

I have thrived on being a student of Zen Master Thich Nhat Hanh for more than thirty years, becoming an OI member, and having breakfast with him in Plum Village, France.

I have thrived on becoming a certified teacher of the enneagram.

I have thrived on serving on the Board of Directors of the Marin AIDS Project and the Advisory Committee of the Institute for Health and Healing.

I have thrived on achieving my Ph. D. in computer science and a successful career in high-tech with five patents to my name.

I have thrived on writing more than 1,000 articles on meditation practices and health and healing on my blogs.

I have thrived on publishing four books and six guided meditations.

I have thrived on creating and leading the **Mindfulness in Healing** sangha (a meditation group) for more than six years.

I have thrived on the wonderful organic fruits and vegetables available in my area and the nearby natural beauty.

I have thrived on the many trips I have taken by myself and with my family.

I have thrived on reconnecting with physics through astronomy, cosmology, and Buddhist thought.

I have thrived on feelings of gratitude and forgiveness and sending loving kindness blessings to people in my life and in the world.

I have thrived on living with cancer for 18+ years utilizing the **Seven Principles of Mindfulness in Healing** for my recovery.

1 INTRODUCTION

Lying still,
Breathing in, breathing out,
Healthy cells grow all by themselves.
I am free of cancer!

Today is June 18, 2014. This is an auspicious day.

On this day in 2009, the *sangha* (meditation group) called **Mindfulness in Healing**[1] began at the Pine Street Clinic in San Anselmo, California. We have been sitting weekly for six straight years with as little as three or four days missed due to illness or holidays. One of us, my partner, Carolyn de Fay, LCSW or I or both have been there almost every week for the past six years.

This sitting group was the result of my efforts to give back to my community after twelve years of living with bladder cancer. It is my way to express the gratitude I felt for all the love and support I experienced during my healing experience from cancer, which began on Super Bowl Sunday in 1997.

I was fortunate enough to have known about alternative medicine – also known as natural, complementary, collaborative or integrative medicine - even before I had cancer.

MICAH'S STORY

My son, Micah, in 1976 at the age of seven was stricken with a grade four, stage four metastatic Wilm's tumor (a cancer of the kidney common in young children) that had spread to his lungs. No one, probably, except me, thought he would survive. He is now 46 and quite a strong and healthy young man.

The key to his survival may have been the use of some of the alternative medical treatments. His surgeon and oncologist had given him up for dead. Even my surgeon said, "We weren't saving many stage fours in those days."

We were totally surprised when his doctors allowed us to use imagery and other alternative medical treatments with him. Micah and I worked together on *mind stories*, guided imagery sessions designed especially for children, from the first day he went into the hospital.

After he got out of the hospital, there were still rounds of chemotherapy and radiation he had to go through. There was also the wonderful Dr. Sheldon Ruderman who continued to do mind stories with Micah for many months.

My son's story was told in two episodes of "In Search of..." with Leonard Nimoy in 1976 and 1980. For more information about Micah's miraculous healing, please check out "Mind Stories Helped Cure Cancer[2]" on **Meditation Practices**[4] website.

STOPPING CANCER IN ITS TRACKS

On Super Bowl Sunday in 1997, I had a tremendous amount of blood in my urine. After a brief stay in the hospital, I was diagnosed with muscle invasive bladder cancer (MBIC). Immediately, I began doing research on the internet and looked in to alternative cancer treatments.

For the next year, I was in the mill of the complex medical establishment. I didn't have the recommended procedure, a radical cystectomy - the complete removal of the bladder, prostate, and lymph nodes.

Instead, our friend, Dr. Sara Huang, MD, the head radiation oncologist at St. Francis Hospital in San Francisco, told me about the Shipley Protocol. This protocol is a bladder sparing protocol that uses a combination of radiation and chemotherapy along with transurethral resection of the bladder tumor (TURBT). It was developed by Dr. William U. Shipley, MD at Harvard University and Massachusetts General Hospital.

During that whole year, I practiced meditation and participated in many different and wonderful alternative medical treatments. These are all well documented in my book, *Stop Cancer in its Tracks: Your Path to Mindfulness in Healing Yourself*[3].

CANCER AGAIN?

In January, 2014, I was diagnosed with a new muscle invasive cancer in my bladder. I call this the 2013 episode because the cancer was discovered but not diagnosed in late 2013.

As before in 1997, the recommended procedure was a radical cystectomy. I was opposed to radical cystectomy then as I am now, only this time there really seemed to be no other choice.

Like before, in 1997, I began doing research and learned that there had been no major changes in the treatment of bladder cancer in past twenty years. So I was out on a limb again, doing my own thing, taking "the road not taken."

I was offered neoadjuvant chemotherapy prior to surgery and decided to try it to postpone the radical cystectomy. I was supposed to have four cycles of chemotherapy lasting twelve weeks and only managed to complete two of them. By the seventh week my creatinine (a measure of kidney function) had gone high and my blood counts had dropped.

Dr. Maxwell Meng, MD, at the University of California San Francisco (UCSF) is now "the go to guy" for bladder cancer. Upon hearing the results of the blood work, he cancelled the rest of the chemotherapy plan and charged me with deciding whether to have the radical cystectomy within the next three to four weeks.

I decided to decline the offer and opted instead for a cystoscopy – a procedure that allows the doctor to look into the bladder through the urethra. I was overjoyed when Dr. Meng said, "I don't see anything that I would want to biopsy." This was a wonderful result.

Ten days later I was notified that I still had cancer in my bladder as determined from the cytology report on the urine sample. This was only surface cancer which is easy to treat.

I think most people would give up at this point and opt for the radical cystectomy. But I was offered a biopsy under anesthesia as an alternative and this is what took place on June 7, 2014.

The results of the biopsy showed that there is no cancer in the muscle of the bladder, but there was carcinoma in situ on the surface. This gives rise to the type of treatment I've done several times already called BCG or Bacillus Calmette-Guerin, an attenuated preparation of a strain of tuberculosis vaccine. The vaccine is instilled into the bladder and causes an immune response. The immune response takes out the cancer along with the bacteria.

This round of six BCG treatments ended at the end of August, 2014. On October 15, I learned that the cytology report after the BCG treatments was benign. **I am once again free of cancer in my bladder**.

Following is valuable information about how you can benefit from the **Seven Principles of Mindfulness in Healing**. Please continue reading.

SEVEN PRINCIPLES OF MINDFULNESS IN HEALING

The seven principles of mindfulness in healing were the underlying principles that guided and continue to guide my well-being through the past forty years or more. I had never explicitly written them down until about two years ago and then I forgot about them until the middle of the 2013 episode.

These principles were implicit in just about everything I did to stop cancer in its tracks and promote my well-being as well as my son's. By writing them down and sharing them with you in this book, **I intend to inspire you to take charge of your own healing experience. My goal is that you learn to be an advocate for your own health care.**

Don't worry if you are not yet willing or able to be your own advocate for medical care. You certainly will gain a lot of new information that will teach you to become your own advocate, or, at least, to know how to find and recognize one that can help you get better faster and more completely.

When you are you own advocate for health care and are deeply involved mentally as well as emotionally and physically, you will be led to investigate the underlying causes of your illness and be informed about your decisions.

I am not telling you to ignore the standard medical treatment in any way. I am suggesting that you take charge of your own medical care so that you can feel better, increase your chances of survival, and learn to make appropriate decisions for your medical care.

We all know that our medical system is complex. It is no longer being run by the Food and Drug Administration (FDA). It is being run by big pharmaceutical companies whose only interest is the bottom line and return on investment for their investors. How many potential cures for cancer have been overlooked because they do not provide enough return on investment to do the necessary evaluations through clinical trials (see below)?

As we move along, there will be many alternatives to the medical system that you may want to investigate. I have tried many of these, and I do feel that many of them have merit under the right circumstances. Just to have them for consideration can lift some of the burden of dealing with a life-threatening situation.

Our first instinct is to follow the advice of our doctors. It takes a lot of courage to think outside the box of standard medical practice. Many people will not want to or be able to do this.

However, if you continue reading, you may be inspired to take up the challenge of being your own advocate for health care. You will be able to use the *Seven Principles of Mindfulness in Healing* as a guide to your medical care. Then you will feel like you own them.

I have written *Seven Principles of Mindfulness in Healing* in order to inspire you, whatever your illness, to **become your own advocate** for health care. I feel that it is important for you to participate in your healing experience and not just roll over and let the medical establishment run over you.

I believe that if you are diagnosed with a serious illness, you should **investigate alternatives**, as I have done and choose the ones that you feel right for you.

I know that it is important for you to **make health-promoting lifestyle changes** to accommodate your new life situation. This may include abstaining from sugar, gluten, meat, dairy and other SAD foods (Standard American Diet) and food substances. This may also include mindful movements and other forms of exercise like Tai Chi and Qi Gong or just walking in nature.

I urge to take on a **daily mindfulness practice** so that you can withdraw yourself into yourself and become aware of what is really going on in your body, feelings, sensations, and mind. I recommend that you follow my blog, **Meditation Practices**[4].

I have often recommended that you **reach out to others**, gather your family and friends to help support you through difficult times. This includes joining support groups like the **Mindfulness in Healing** sangha or one specifically oriented to what ails you.

I have found **creating my own team of medical practitioners** who know both Eastern and Western methods indispensable for my healing. They have pointed me in the right directions over the past 18 years.

I propose that when you are ready, you should **give back to the community** that supported you during your recovery period. This will give you the same sense of joy I experience in leading the **Mindfulness in Healing** sangha.

These, in a nutshell, are the seven principles of mindfulness in healing.

2 SEVEN PRINCIPLES OF MINDFULNESS IN HEALING

The *Seven Principles of Mindfulness in Healing* are presented in subsequent chapters, with illustrations from my healing experiences and others. We begin with a brief summary of each principle.

The Seven Principles of
Mindfulness in Healing

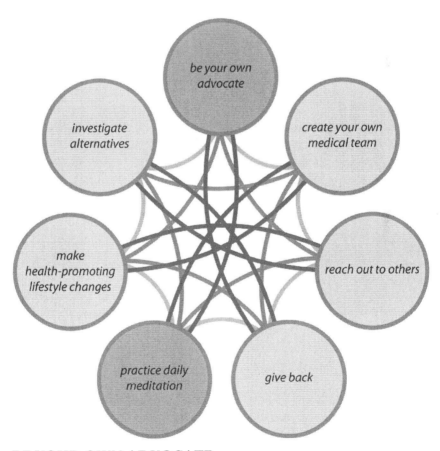

BE YOUR OWN ADVOCATE

Become an advocate for your own health care. This means to take charge of your own health care and not leave everything up to the doctors. It is fine to listen to them and understand what they are asking you to do.

However, you must take responsibility for your own healing by participating, being actively involved, and being willing to explore possibilities. Getting second and third opinions may help.

Talking to friends and relatives who are knowledgeable about health matters can also help. Most of all, unless you have extreme circumstances, take a few days to think things over.

The principle to be your own advocate is one of two foundational principles of mindfulness in healing, the other being practice daily meditation. Without adopting this principle, it is difficult to get motivated to investigate alternatives and make health-promoting lifestyle changes.

INVESTIGATE ALTERNATIVES

Investigate alternatives and complementary healing methods to enhance your healing experience. Many alternative treatments can relieve a lot of stress and suffering just by participating in them.

To name a few, we have found that acupuncture, massage, body work, Qi Gong, yoga and other movement therapies, meditation, guided imagery, and creative expression can really help.

In participating in these kinds of activities, you are encouraged to do as much or as little as you feel comfortable doing.

MAKE HEALTH-PROMOTING LIFESTYLE CHANGES

Find out about the best possible lifestyle changes in diet, nutrition, supplements, and exercise that can improve your overall health. Lifestyle changes can be one of the most important factors for your recovery.

Studies at the University of Massachusetts in the Mindfulness Based Stress Reduction program over the past 33 years have shown that opting for a vegetarian diet along with yoga and meditation practice can reduce symptoms and even help produce unexpected cures.

Dr. Dean Ornish has proven that the right kind of diet and exercise can reverse heart disease and reduce the effects of prostate cancer.

PRACTICE DAILY MEDITATION

Develop a daily meditation practice to cope with changes in

physical, emotional, mental, and spiritual states with equanimity. One of the best things you can do for yourself is to have a daily meditation practice. It is possible to begin with just nine minutes a day and build up to 30 minutes or more.

Practice daily meditation is the second of the foundational principles of mindfulness in healing. While, for some people, this may not seem to be as important as the principle to be your own advocate, it really is. The reason for this is that meditation provides you with a calm, clear mind and reduces stress so that you can weigh your alternatives and make desirable decisions for you healthcare.

REACH OUT TO OTHERS

Gather your family and friends for support and find an appropriate support group. We have found that the support of family and friends is extremely important and beneficial.

In addition, taking part in organized support groups helps everyone. Dr. Daniel Goleman has reported in his books that a significant amount of healing can be gained from participation in support groups. Participating in such groups can improve longevity by as much as 40 percent.

CREATE YOUR OWN MEDICAL TEAM

Find a healing professional who knows about your standard medical treatment plan and complementary medicine to help manage your well-being. Most people have only their primary physician or surgeon to rely on for medical care. Your primary doctor may be able to fulfill this role.

While this may be adequate in many circumstances, we have found it beneficial to converse and rely on advice from other competent practitioners. They can give you a perspective that is "outside the box" of standard medical practice.

You may wish to consult an acupuncturist, naturopath, chiropractor, doctor of Chinese medicine and herbs, or a homeopath to be your medical advisor.

GIVE BACK TO YOUR COMMUNITY

Give back to your community when the time is right. Your community supports your healing efforts and you will experience a lot of joy when you feel comfortable contributing to the benefit of others.

HOW TO USE THIS BOOK

These principles are easy to adapt to just about any lifestyle. Most likely, you'll have to make some adjustments, however.

The first time through, you might want to read the introductory section of each chapter, saving the details for when you are in need of them. For example, in Chapter 4 (**Investigate Alternatives**) there is an introduction to alternative medical practices which precedes the subchapter on Homeopathy. You might want to read just the introductory text on your first pass through.

Some chapters don't have subchapters. These should be read to completion during your first pass through. If you don't read anything else, be sure to read the section on **The Cancer Diet** in Chapter 5.

However, it is your choice on how you want to use this book. You may at least want to see what the subchapters contain before you move on. The Table of Contents can give you a good idea about this.

Taking on the attitude of becoming your own advocate for health care is an important way to begin. It is considered the entry point to the *Seven Principles of Mindfulness in Healing*, and probably really essential. Without this attitude, it can be difficult to embrace the other principles.

Each one is valuable in its own right and they all work together to enhance your life and create the best possible mindset for a complete recovery. They don't have to be undertaken in any specific order.

For example, exploring alternative and complementary care (i.e., integrative medicine, does not require a healing professional that is familiar with both standard medical practices and integrative medicine, but in my experience, having Michael Broffman at the Pine Street Clinic as my healing professional and guide through the complex cancer system was a tremendous benefit.

I have found that my mindfulness practices have helped me integrate all seven of the principles of mindfulness in healing. I used many different mindfulness practices at various stages in my healing process.

One of the turning points occurred on the Vernal Equinox of 1997. I had a very powerful guided imagery session which served as the path for healing and inspiration to continue practicing. This imagery session was also the motivation for the title of *Stop Cancer in its Tracks: Your Path to Mindfulness in Healing Yourself*[3] and the cover image.

Other practices included sitting meditation, walking meditation, mindful movements, dance, creative writing and drawing, and meditation in bed when I couldn't do anything else. Being on retreat with Zen Master Thich Nhat Hanh came at a perfect time and provided me with a lot of love and support at a time when it was badly needed.

As I approach my nineteenth year of living with cancer, I find that meditation practices keep me on track with my healing experience and provide me with a refuge from fear, doubt, uncertainty, and worry. I feel that they are strong enough to help me embrace any situation I find myself in with regard to cancer and health issues.

Returning to my true home – my mindfulness of the present moment – relieves the stress of having to think about consequences, obstacles, and worst case scenarios. I stay on top of my feelings and this helps keep my family from feeling morose about my situation.

3 BE YOUR OWN ADVOCATE

The first principle of mindfulness in healing is to be your own advocate. As much as the doctors know, they don't live inside your skin and they really don't know for sure whether the treatment they are offering is best or even right for you.

There is a tremendous gap between what the doctors know and how they perceive you will receive the information. You have to make it clear to them that you are not going to be an easy patient. You are going to stand up for your rights and take charge of your medical care.

By reading this book, **you will to learn to take charge of your medical care**. Ask a lot of questions. Research your disease on the internet and in the library. Talk to people who have the same disease. Share your feelings openly with your family and friends. Don't go into hibernation.

You may even want to get a second or third opinion. Your research should provide you with a couple of references, if your standard medical treatment doctor doesn't know or want to refer you.

If your situation does not require immediate hospitalization (like mine did in 1997), take a few days to think about things and talk things over. Try to get as much information as you can from people you know. Find out if there is anyone in your area that has the same condition and try to contact them.

But most of all, investigate alternative medical treatments that can make you feel comfortable and make your life much easier in the long run. For example, you might try massage, acupuncture, or guided imagery. These will be covered in the next chapter.

Investigate lifestyle changes that can support your healing experience. What changes can you make to your diet to ease the burden of your digestive track? What supplements can you take to boost your immune system? What exercises are you able to do, even at this time? Walking is a very good one.

When you get diagnosed with a life-threatening illness, it can be a shock to your system. Your body is already probably experiencing some symptoms. Either you have some physical pain or discomfort or both. At least, you have been informed that you have a problem.

The effect on your emotions can be much more drastic. You are probably wondering, "How can this happen to me?" At times, you may feel like jumping off the Golden Gate Bridge. You may feel like running away and not dealing with anything. You may feel like doing physical harm to someone, maybe the doctor who gave you the news.

None of these solutions will actually work very well if at all. Yet, you have to deal with your feelings in some manner. Hopefully, your doctor, spouse, or close friend will provide you with some immediate support and you can carry on investigating your options.

Perhaps you can join a support group to discuss your thoughts, feelings, fears and anxieties with other people in the same or similar situation.

Then, this news affects your mental state as well. You begin to have all sorts of visions about what is going to happen to you and your life. You think you want to try anything, but when it gets right down to it, you just want to follow the doctor's orders and be done with it.

The problem is, no one has prepared you for news of this kind. You may have had an inclination that something bad was happening, but you were too afraid to really confront it. Instead, you relied on your doctor to help.

There is a practical way to overcome all of this, depending on how deeply you want to pursue you symptoms prior to and after consulting with you primary care physician. You can do the type of research I did when I first noticed that I had urine in my blood! I spent hours on the computer investigating the symptoms, causes, and treatments for what turned out to be bladder cancer.

By the time I got to see my doctor to receive the information, I was able to point to a printout I brought with me showing the information he was poised to tell me. My wife and four friends, one a medical doctor (Dr. Marty Rossman, MD), came with me for support. This made the diagnosis much easier to take.

You can make a list of questions to ask your doctor. They should be formulated around your major concerns. You can use some or all of these questions as you like:

- Will I need surgery?
- What are the preoperative considerations? Medical? Legal? Financial?

- What, exactly, are you going to do?
- What, exactly, are you going to remove?
- How long will the hospital stay be?
- How long is the recovery period at home?
- What complications may arise? What complications have you seen with my condition?
- What activities can I do and when?
- What will my life be like after I recover?
- What kind of follow-up is required?
- How can I prevent infection?
- Will I need chemotherapy (if it is cancer)?
  - What kind of chemotherapy?
  - What drugs will be used?
  - What are the side effects?
  - How are they handled?
  - How will chemo affect my longevity?
  - Will it be before or after surgery? Radiation?
  - Will I experience neuropathy? How serious will it be? What can I do for it?
- Will I need radiation therapy (if it is cancer)?
  - What kind of radiation?
  - What drugs or tracers will be used?
  - What are the side effects?
  - How are they handled?
  - How will radiation affect my longevity?
  - Will it be before or after surgery? Chemotherapy?
  - What can I use to reduce the effects of burning?
- What caused my illness?
- What are the stage and grade (if it is cancer)?
- Is it fast growing?
- What is my life expectancy?
- What are the chances of recurrence?
- How long do I have before I must take action?
- Are there any other courses of treatment?
- What is your success rate with this kind of illness?
- What is the average success rate with this kind of illness?

- What should my diet be like before, during and after treatment?
- Is there something about the treatment that you are unwilling to tell me?
- What would you do if this happened to you?

Perhaps the two most important questions are the last two! Doctors may tell you one thing that they overlooked and you may be able to tell from their facial expressions what they really mean, especially in response to the last question.

Remember, being your own advocate for medical treatment also means listening to your doctor, but not necessarily agreeing with him. Getting second and third opinions are helpful, if you feel up to it.

I found it extremely beneficial to record all my consultations with medical practitioners. iPhones make this very easy to do and you can refer to them later if necessary. Recordings make a wonderful, unbiased listener.

4 INVESTIGATE ALTERNATIVES

No matter what is wrong with you, there is bound to be something useful "outside the box" of standard medical treatment that can bring you a little or a lot of relief. In fact, there are so many alternative treatments that they could be the subject of a book all by themselves.

What I am going to do here is to describe what I consider to be the best ones, along with examples from my life and the lives of others and how they will benefit you. In addition, I am going to tell you about the different kinds of practitioners and what kinds of services they offer.

HOMEOPATHY

I'm starting with homeopathy because there was a radical change between 1997 and 2014. Also, Dr. Roger Morrison, MD, was the first person we saw outside of Dr. Marty Rossman, MD, that we talked to after the initial hospital stay in 1997.

Homeopathy is a holistic, non-invasive medical system which treats the whole human being (and animals) with highly diluted substances. These come mostly in the form of pellets which can be the size of a period (.) or the small letter "O" (o).

The goal of homeopathy is to trigger the body's natural system of healing. Substances are recommended on the basis of symptoms. Therefore, homeopaths take an extra-long time evaluating you and your medical history. When was the last time a doctor spent more than 7½ minutes with you?

Benefits of Homeopathy

You can benefit from homeopathy even if you are pregnant or nursing. Your young children can also benefit, just like mine did.

Homeopathic remedies do not interfere with the medicine you are taking and it is completely safe and harmless as long as you follow the instructions of your practitioner. They almost always produce no symptoms and they can be used for chronic as well as acute conditions.

Homeopathic doctors work on an individual basis. You'll have to fill out a long form, and answer a lot of questions, but your treatment is totally individualized.

You'll be happy to know that homeopathic remedies are usually quite inexpensive relative to medicines from the big pharmaceutical companies and often don't expire.

Dr. Roger Morrison, MD

When my girls were small, we consulted Dr. Morrison quite frequently. One memorable example was when my youngest had bulging ear infections and the pediatrician wanted to install tubes in her ears. We took Jessica to Roger, and the remedy he gave her worked the same day. She never needed tubes in her ears.

In 1997, Roger had no magic bullet for bladder cancer. Homeopathy, at that time, was not able to do anything directly with cancer other than to prescribe what is called a "constitutional remedy."

I was encouraged by one of my closest friends to go see Roger in 2014. Being a retired homeopathic practitioner herself, and having collaborated with Roger on his book, she knew of a remedy for cancer that was developed by Dr. A. U. Ramkrishnan in India. This time, Roger had an answer.

He offered me a remedy which is taken in a very strange way. I've been doing it now for more than a year and I still think it's strange.

There are two remedies taken every day on alternate weeks. Since both remedies come in period-sized pellets, I need to use about twenty of them from each remedy. I start the week of with the twenty pellets of *conium* diluted in eleven teaspoons of filtered or distilled water plus one-half and inch of extra water in a jar. I then proceed to take a teaspoon every ten to fifteen minutes until I have taken ten teaspoons of the remedy and add ten more teaspoons of water back in the jar at the end. On the seventh day, I take an extra spoonful and throw out the rest. On the next day and for the next week, I do the same for *carcinosin*. This whole procedure goes on for about a year. We'll see what the results are like.

FAITH HEALING AND SHAMANISM

Nicholi Levachov

I've chosen this topic as the second one to report on because after visiting Dr. Morrison that day in 1997, we drove to San Francisco to meet Nicholi Levaschov. He struck me as a powerful faith healer. He used his hands to make circles around the area of my bladder and the healing energy was palpable. I decided not to engage him, even though I could feel his energy quite viscerally. His rates far exceeded my budget and expectations.

Father Eli

The first shaman I encountered in my life was Father Eli. I met him in a spiritual bookstore in Evanston, Illinois in 1972. He was giving a series of lectures on the history and transmission of his wisdom tradition.

I was captivated by his voice and entranced by his stories. They say that all great shamans and teachers have great stories, and Father Eli was no exception. By the summer of 1973, I was convinced that attending his retreat center in the Ozark Mountains of Arkansas was the right thing to do.

That summer, I learned how to train people to put themselves in a deep meditative state using relaxation and visualization. My **Guided Meditations** (see Chapter 11) follow the same method I learned from Father Eli all those years ago. This training carried forward to the time when my son had cancer, and I could teach him how to do *mind stories* to help him heal, as reported in Chapter 1.

A few months prior to meeting Father Eli, I had taken the Silva Mind Control course. When I recognized components of Father Eli's teaching being identical to what I learned from the Silva Method, I asked him, "This is so much like Silva Mind Control."

His response was, "It better be. Jose Silva was one of my students!"

I later learned that Dr. Sheldon Ruderman, Micah's mentor and guide, was trained by Carl Simonton and that the Simontons were students of Jose Silva. Completing this circle made me feel well validated.

Don Alejandro

I have joined faith healing with laying on of the hands and shamanism because they are all closely related. In 1997, and later in 2010, I had several experiences with shamans. The first shaman I saw was about two and one-half months after seeing Roger. He was a Peruvian named Don Alejandro. I had to talk to him through an interpreter. Nonetheless, we got some valuable healing and information.

I went in with a handful of questions. He told me that the bladder cancer was hereditary and that I would be healed but it would take some time.

After discussing my treatment plan, he began chanting in an unrecognizable language. This was followed by his laying on of his hands on my bladder area. This part of the treatment was really amazing!

The lessons I learned from this provided me with the strong desire to make sure I would recover. I learned that I had to let go of my defenses and allow his healing energy to penetrate into my bladder. By maintaining my awareness of breathing, I was also able to learn how to embrace the pain that some of his manipulations caused me. The pain was actually a part of the healing process.

Gabrielle Roth

Gabrielle Roth was an American shaman who started an international organization based on her book, *The Five Rhythms*. The five rhythms include flowing, staccato, chaos, lyrical, and stillness. I believe these were inspired by the chaotic meditation taught by Bhagwan Shree Rajneesh (Osho).

I spent one evening with her in 1997 after being out of touch for many years. Reconnecting with her was wonderful and now I have connected with many people who practice the five rhythms weekly.

For a little more than a year before the time my son had cancer in 1976, I spent a lot of time with Gabrielle. We danced and celebrated our connection with Rajneesh. One winter night, we gathered 250 people for a celebration honoring him.

Eric Vormanns

Eric Vormanns is a West African shaman and energy healer who I met in 1997. This man told me that the cancer would eventually go away, and that I wasn't activating my full potential. I wasn't doing what I came in this life to do.

He thought that I should be writing, teaching, and practicing in the areas of mindfulness in healing and meditation. Now, with the publication of this book, my work on the **Meditation Practices** website[4], and my other books and guided meditations, I am beginning to live up to my potential.

What's in it for You

When you visit a shaman, it is best to have a set of questions that you want to ask. The shaman may not know about standard medical practice, but they can tune into your body, emotions and metal state to determine what is best for you.

I advise you to be prepared for anything that happens. I have heard stories of miracles that take place at the hand of a shaman. Life-changing insights can come to you in a single moment while being treated. Be open, relax, and take your experience just as it is.

ACUPUNCTURE

Acupuncture is an ancient Chinese medical practice based on the stimulation of various points on the body along meridians through which energy flows. The stimulation is done by needles, pressure, heat, and other techniques.

Benefits of Acupuncture

When acupuncture is performed correctly, it is totally safe, although you may experience some discomfort from time to time. There are very few side effects and it can be very effective when combined with other treatment.

As you'll see in the next sections, it can help to control pain and you may respond to acupuncture if you have difficulty with pain medication.

Acupuncture can help you unblock some of your energy from where it is being held. Like the effect of Dr. Vu's (see below) treatment on my back, you may experience a release of substantial proportions when you go in for acupuncture treatments.

Dr. Marty Rossman, MD

Dr. Marty Rossman, MD is a medical doctor, acupuncturist, author, and teacher of guided imagery. In fact, he founded the Academy for Guided Imagery and trained thousands of practitioners. One of them, Leslie Davenport became my therapist and led me in life changing guided imagery sessions. There will be more about guided imagery later in this chapter.

My first session of acupuncture with Marty had an unsuspected emotional impact on me. Marty had been present with me when Dr. Neuwirth pronounced my first diagnosis of bladder cancer. He also visited me in the hospital that first day.

Having a friend and feeling his love during the acupuncture sessions during the first and recent episodes made a huge difference.

During the 2013 episode, Marty treated me before each chemotherapy session. The effects were subtle and helped reduce the impact of the chemotherapy.

Dr. Van Vu

Soon after I received my diagnosis I experienced extreme back pain. I could barely walk. Luckily, Dr. Van Vu, MD, a Vietnamese Buddhist acupuncturist and medical doctor was seeing patients in Mill Valley that day. He stuck a few needles in my back and I walked out of the office without any residual pain.

MASSAGE AND BODY WORK

Massage is just about everyone's favorite alternative treatment. It certainly is one of mine, and it usually feels good. Sometimes, massage therapists go a little overboard and cause some pain, but it is usually short lived. In many cases this pain "hurts good!"

Body work is slightly different from massage, and the distinction is rather difficult to define. I consider massage to be more about feeling good and less about healing. With body work, the goal is more about healing along with feeling good.

If you don't like this distinction, simply ignore it. You won't hurt my feelings.

Benefits of Massage and Body Work

In most cases, massage increases circulation and enhances the immune system. It promotes the functioning of the nervous system and reduces high blood pressure.

A good masseuse can relieve a lot of pain and reduce muscle tension. You will almost always feel good after a massage and your mood will be uplifted. It can help to improve reasoning and job performance. This is why places like Google have full-time massage personnel.

Massage can also have a positive effect on cancer, fibromyalgia, arthritis, diabetes, and migraine headaches.

Elyse, Gail and Others

I had many wonderful massages from both Elyse and Gail during the early years of living with bladder cancer. In every massage, I felt relaxed and comfortable. I found them all to be healing in unique ways each time.

In conjunction with chemotherapy, California Cancer Care also offered massages for free. Naturally I took advantage of these offers.

I have also had wonderful massages in my hospital room and while receiving chemotherapy.

Jessica Zerr

Jessica Zerr was one of my daughter's yoga teachers and she also does body work. In my first session with her, she did craniosacral work and I was impressed. This was about a year before the beginning of the 2013 episode.

I have been seeing Jessica for treatments about three times a month. I'd prefer to do it more often, but she was quite booked up and has now moved to Philadelphia.

Her treatment specialties are quite hard to describe. Sometimes she works on the organs in my chest and abdomen. You can't believe how good this feels. It was especially useful when I was trying to get rid of the toxic effects of chemotherapy.

At other times, she'll work on the lymphatic system and you can experience the fresh energy generated from the cleansing. She also does tissue manipulation to realign various parts of my body.

I never know what to expect because she treats the whole body. She is a magnificent healer with total presence and focused energy.

GUIDED IMAGERY

Guided imagery is a process which involves all the senses as well as focused imagination to help you tune into whatever problem or symptom you are dealing with. It works well through the mind-body connection to reach deep inside of you to bring out your true feelings and sensations about your situation.

Ordinarily, you work with a guided imagery professional who could also be your therapist or your doctor. At other times, you can listen to guided imagery recordings or work on your own and gain almost the same benefit as working with a therapist or doctor.

Benefits of Guided Imagery

Guided imagery promotes and relies on deep relaxation; the deeper the relaxation, the better the results. Deep relaxation also helps to lower blood pressure.

Deep relaxation potentiates your ability to visualize and has several benefits on its own. You are actually much better at visualization then you think you are.

One of the most significant benefits is the reduction of problems related to stress. It stimulates the relaxation response, first researched by Dr. Herbert Benson, MD of Harvard University, but really as old as the Vedas (ancient Hindu writings) or older.

In addition, it helps to reach goals, reduce weight, relieve symptoms, alleviate pain, control anger, and helps you sleep (see Chapter 11). I can't tell you how many times I've fallen asleep in the middle of a self-guided imagery session!

Guided imagery may help increase your creativity, performance, and learning abilities. It can also help you learn to control your emotions and thoughts, which can lead to better health, improved attitudes, and a sense of well-being.

With guided imagery and guided meditation you can learn to breathe deeply into and out of your abdomen; bring your attention into your breath, body and feelings; create a relaxing scene for you to return to at will; and scan your body to achieve a state of total relaxation as well as many other benefits.

Leslie Davenport

Probably the most improvement that I experienced in 1997 was the result of a guided imagery session which took place on the vernal equinox. I had several sessions with her prior to this one. At that time of the year I am often reminded of a Zen poem which goes like this:

> *Sitting quietly,*
> *Doing nothing,*
> *Spring comes*
> *And the grass grows by itself.*

During the guided imagery session, I saw myself walking down a grassy hill with a wandering dirt path. I was saying to my wife, whose hand I was holding, "It's all downhill from here!" I was reminded of Robert Frost's famous poem, *The Road Not Taken*.

The complete text of Robert Frost's poem, *The Road Not Taken*, is:

> *Two roads diverged in a yellow wood,*
> *And sorry I could not travel both*
> *And be one traveler, long I stood*
> *And looked down one as far as I could*
> *To where it bent in the undergrowth;*
> *Then took the other, as just as fair,*
> *And having perhaps the better claim,*
> *Because it was grassy and wanted wear;*
> *Though as for that the passing there*
> *Had worn them really about the same,*
> *And both that morning equally lay*
> *In leaves no step had trodden black.*
> *Oh, I kept the first for another day!*
> *Yet knowing how way leads on to way,*
> *I doubted if I should ever come back.*
> *I shall be telling this with a sigh*
> *Somewhere ages and ages hence:*
> *Two roads diverged in a wood, and I --*
> *I took the one less traveled by,*
> *And that has made all the difference.*

I took the road less travelled by not following the gold standard of medical treatment for bladder cancer, and recognizing this led me into a state of bliss that was extremely healing. I knew then, as I know now, that I took the right path to recovery.

I took the image of the strong, vibrant, healthy grass, growing by itself as a metaphor for going deep into my bladder for healing and comfort. I constructed my own poem that you saw in Chapter 1:

> *Lying still,*
> *Breathing in, breathing out*

Healthy cells grow all by themselves.
I am free of cancer!

I suspect that the deep experience of bliss that was directed towards my ailing bladder had a profound effect on my healing process. I also suspect that this is a valuable lesson that you can use, so long as you are able to get far enough away from your pain and suffering into a state of bliss.

HYPERBARIC OXYGEN THERAPY

You probably haven't heard of hyperbaric oxygen therapy unless you are a sports buff and have learned that Novak Djokovic (#1 tennis player), Terrell Owens (American football player), Nick Anderson (basketball player), John Smoltz (baseball player), and many other athletes have purchased hyperbaric oxygen chambers for their own personal use.

So that's the clue – hyperbaric oxygen therapy is administered in a hyperbaric oxygen chamber in which additional oxygen is introduced to increase the oxygen content in a pressurized chamber up to four times the normal amount in air. This greatly increases the oxygenation of organs, tissues, and body fluids. The pressure in the chamber allows for much greater absorption of the oxygen provided.

Dr. Geoffry Saft, DC says,

In the USA, the situation stands in marked contrast with many other countries where HBOT [hyperbaric oxygen therapy] is used for a much wider range of conditions. There are over 60 medical conditions being treated worldwide, using HBOT. Multiple Sclerosis patients have banded together in Britain to create their own network of Hyperbaric Chambers. Centers in China treat more than 100,000 patients each year for a multitude of medical conditions. In France Germany, and Japan, Hyperbaric Oxygen Therapy is also a much-used therapy, in contrast to the United States.

According to Dr. Saft, the following conditions respond well to hyperbaric oxygen therapy: stroke, autism, ADD / ADHD, fibromyalgia, Alzheimer's, memory loss, A. L. S., R. S. D., wounds, multiple sclerosis, cerebral palsy, head injuries, migraines, Parkinson's disease, insomnia, Crohn's disease, diabetes, Lyme disease, AIDS, chemical sensitivities, chronic fatigue syndrome, brain damage, cancer, and heart disease. It is also good for pre- and post-surgery as was well as in detoxification programs.

During the time of BCG treatments in 2010, Dr. Saft offered me many treatments of hyperbaric oxygen therapy. The results were quite beneficial and I probably fell asleep each time I was in the chamber. It is a wonderful time to bring in your iPhone or MP3 player and listen to a guided meditation.

AYURVEDA

Ayurveda is the medicine of ancient India. It has its roots in the Vedas, some of the first written documents in human history. It is still practiced today.

I am especially proud of my daughter, Rachael, who is a yoga teacher and an Ayurveda practitioner.

During 2014, I had three wonderful experiences with Ayurveda. The first was a puja – a ceremony to celebrate the participation of many people in the Ayurveda training with Dr. Sarita Shrestha, OB/GYN.

Dr. Shrestha is Nepal's first female Ayurvedic physician and OB/GYN. She is the only known female doctor currently teaching in the United States, and the founder of the Deva Ma Ayurveda Rural Hospital in Sipadole, Nepal.

The second experience was my one-on-one consultation with Dr. Shrestha. She gave me advice on diet, meditation, and body work. She said I should eat no yogurt and fewer nuts, especially cashews. Also I should try to chant the *Mahamrityunjaya Mantra* at least eleven times before going to bed. Parts of the mantra play in my mind, especially when I feel the least bit tense or anxious.

The third experience was an Ayurvedic treatment with Simone de Winter at Marin Ayuveda. I wrote, "I was treated to a wonderful Ayurveda treatment by my three children. It was a birthday present that I'll remember for a long time, especially when I have more treatments like this one. They set me up with Simone for a full body massage (*abhyanga*), oil on forehead (*shirodhara*), domes filled with oil on the kidneys (*basti*), and a steam tent (*swedana*). There were many minutes when my breathing slowed down to almost a complete stop. The whole experience was amazing."

IMMUNOTHERAPY AND OFF LABEL TREATMENTS

In my initial consultation with Michael Broffman when the 2013 episode began, we talked about immunotherapy and what he called "off label" treatments.

Immunotherapy is a treatment that utilizes your own immune system to cause a cure. As reported above, the BCG treatments I had were a form of immunotherapy. In fact, I have been told by Dr. Johanna Olweus, MD, a distinguished immunotherapy researcher at Oslo University that BCG was probably the first and continues to be the best performing type of immunotherapy.

Off label treatments are a class of non-standard treatments that have the blessing of the FDA, but are not mainstream. You'll see some examples below.

Michael's recommendation was to read about and investigate these interventions until we discussed them in more detail.

But first, an interesting story...

Euphorbia Peplus

Have you ever had a skin lesion that looked suspicious? Did you go to your dermatologist to have it burned off with liquid nitrogen or removed with Mohs surgery?

Mohs surgery is a procedure to remove skin cancers with microscopic control of the margins. You have to wait between successive removals of the tissue in the affected area for the lab to determine whether or not all the cancer cells have been removed.

I had a squamous cell carcinoma on my right temple about two years ago. I was scheduled for Mohs surgery and told my friend about it. He asked me if I had heard of euphorbia peplus – a common form of milkweed.

I had not heard of it, but he had some growing in his yard. He said that the plant had been used for three thousand years in Europe and Australia.

On a Friday afternoon, I went into his back yard and picked some milkweed. I broke open a small stalk and put the sap on my wound.

There was almost an immediate reaction. I had placed a small amount on the upper part of my right cheek and felt the toxic effects of the sap. Then I dabbed the healed biopsy site with a tiny bit of the sap and felt it sting. I was not intimidated by the pain and put another dab on later that evening.

The next morning, I needed a bandage over the area again and didn't think about it too much until Monday afternoon, when I noticed that the new scab was gone and the whole lesion seemed smaller.

On Tuesday evening, I discovered that the lesion had practically disappeared. From its beginning almost three years ago, it appeared as a round growth with activity in the middle – something like a crater on a tiny scale. That night, all that was left was the tiny center.

To clarify, the outer rim may have had a diameter of about 3-4 mm. The inner crater had a diameter of about 1-1.5 mm. Now the outer rim was gone and the crater was flattened, slightly red, and no bigger than a millimeter.

I went into the dermatology office the next day, fully expecting nothing to be done. I felt confident that the milkweed cure for skin cancer actually worked.

When the person at the desk wanted me to sign a document releasing the dermatology group for consequences of the surgery, I noticed a statement that I had been told all the alternatives. This was a red flag to me, so I asked what these alternatives were.

I was led into a treatment room where Dr. Holly Christman was going to meet me and discuss the alternatives. When she came in, she said that for squamous cell carcinoma, there were none. I asked her about radiation and she told me that radiation is recommended only in cases where surgery is not an option. The radiation treatment lasts from four to six weeks and takes 15 minutes each day.

This was not a viable option, considering all the radiation I had experienced during the 1997 episode.

When she saw the size of the growth, she told me that there could be cancer cells underneath. When I told her that I had applied euphorbia peplus to the skin cancer, she seemed a little perplexed and wanted Dr. Scully, my doctor, to see it.

Dr. Scully came into the treatment room, and after appropriate greetings, I took out my iPhone, opened the email for euphorbia peplus, followed the link to the Wikipedia page, and showed her that the active ingredient was ingenol mebutate. This sparked an enthusiastic response during which she started to tell me about some exciting new topical drugs to treat skin cancer.

She left the room, wanting to get the information about the new skin cancer treatments. She also wanted to look at the slides of the squamous cell carcinoma that she took three week prior. I also wanted to look at the slides.

When she came back, she gave me an information brochure of a company that had made a gel of ingenol mebutate that was approved for treatment of actinic keratosis, but not for squamous cell or basal cell carcinoma.

After considering the size of the site and the superficial nature of the skin cancer, she concluded that we didn't have to do anything that day and we should keep a watchful eye on the site.

Thanks to my friend and milkweed (euphorbia peplus), I left the office having saved taxpayers and Medicare a bundle of money.

I felt a sense of euphorbia, oops, I mean euphoria for the rest of the day. My mindfulness, intuition, and willingness to try an alternative therapy ruled the day.

By the way, the commercial product with the active ingredient, ingenol mebutate sells for upwards of $750 for a 1 oz. tube that is a one percent solution. It takes many applications of this costly medicine to have the same effect as the euphorbia peplus sap itself.

Perhaps the reaction one gets when you place a drop of euphorbia peplus sap on a wound is actually an immune response. Supposedly, the sap triggers this response because the cancerous cells are growing more quickly than normal cells.

GcMAF

In my opinion, the GcMAF (Gc protein macrophage activation factor) protocol is the most promising of the immunotherapies that Michael recommended. I got so far as to enquire how much it would cost and what the probable benefits would be.

GcMAF is a human protein and it is used as a replacement therapy for those who don't produce it. It helps reset the immune system to its normal, healthy state.

GcMAF was developed by Dr. Nobuto Yamamoto, MD in Japan. He kept it under wraps for more than 20 years in order to convince himself that it helped in the best case and did no harm in the worst case.

Michael Broffman has been following his research and development for many years. He has visited Dr. Yamamoto and tried to get him to release it for common use.

Today, GcMAF is available in three places in the European Union as well as in Japan. Unfortunately, there is conflict between these suppliers and I found it difficult to decide where to purchase it.

If you are going to investigate one thing in this section, I recommend it be GcMAF.

Recchia Protocol

The Recchia protocol consists of very low doses of IL-2 plus retinoic acid. IL-2 is interleukin 2 – a type of cytokine signaling molecule in the immune system. Dr. Francesco Recchia, MD has reported tremendous success with patients who could not tolerate high doses of IL-2 alone. The Recchia protocol increases the number and supposedly the activity of natural killer cells and decreases the level of endothelial growth factor.

This protocol is particularly attractive to people with stage four (metastatic) cancers. It has helped prolong their lives. The cost of treatment is very inexpensive compared to traditional methods.

DCA

DCA is dichloroacetic acid. In reality the acid is a liquid and researchers used the salt, sodium dichloroacetate. We are warned not to use the acid because it is corrosive.

It has been shown to slow the growth of certain types of tumors in animal studies, but the evidence does not support the use of DCA for the treatment of cancer at this time.

DCA turns on the mitochondria of cancer cells, encouraging them to commit cellular suicide (apoptosis) like normal cells. Cancer cells normally shut down the mitochondria so they can proliferate at will.

You can purchase DCA from suppliers in Canada. Your starting dose should be 5mg/kilo of body weight.

I have not tried this form of treatment yet, but it is one of the highest on my list of possibilities.

Metformin

Cancer cells survive on sugar in the form of glucose. The more glucose in your system, the faster the cancer will grow. You'll learn much more about this later.

Metformin is a drug for the treatment of diabetes, but Michael Broffman thought that it is good for cancer. The purpose is to keep the blood sugar levels down to the low 80s so as not to feed the cancer cells. He recommends 250 mg twice a day.

You will need a prescription to use metformin. I have not tried it.

There are now some indications that insulin use, which also lowers the blood sugar levels, along with chemotherapy is beneficial. This is called Insulin Potentiation Therapy or IPT. IPT has been used in other chronic diseases besides cancer.

The idea is that cancer cells have a great affinity for insulin and therefore it can be used as a Trojan horse to get the chemotherapy into the cancer cells. Since more chemotherapy is getting to the cancer cells, a lower dose of chemotherapy can be used.

So far, there are no clinical trials yet, but some practitioners have had great success. This is definitely a treatment option for people with stage four cancers when everything else has failed.

Tetrathiomolybdate

Tetrathiomolybdate is a prescription drug used in copper reduction therapy. Researchers at the University of Michigan hypothesized that tetrathiomolybdate would help achieve and maintain a mild copper deficiency to deter metastatic solid tumors from generating more blood vessels.

Technically, tetrathiomolybdate is an anticopper and antiangiogenic agent. The recommended dose is 20 mg three times a day with meals and 60 mg on an empty stomach at bedtime. The goal is to bring the ceruloplasmin serum levels (an indication of the amount of copper in the blood) to 20% of the baseline of ceruloplasmin (a number somewhere between 10 and 20).

Once again, I have not done much more than to look into the benefits of tetrathiomolybdate. You may be more included to investigate it further.

Naltrexone

Naltrexone is another prescription drug that has been approved in low doses to help those with HIV/AIDS, cancer, autoimmune diseases, and central nervous system disorders.

Naltrexone boosts the immune system and activates the body's own natural defenses. As I understand, it operates by blocking opioid receptors, thereby allowing an uptake of endorphins and enkephalin levels. This possibly works directly on the cancer cells' opioid receptors.

Michael's recommended dose is 4.5 mg daily. I have only researched naltrexone at the point.

GENETIC INTERVENTIONS

This is a subject that I know very little about. Michael Broffman recommended that I look into whether or not I express certain genes, indicated below. If so, there may be certain treatments that are indicated due to their targeting the genes in question.

Genetic testing is still in its infancy as far as testing for markers for drug selection is concerned. One study used whole-genome sequencing to investigate the genetic basis for long-term remission in a patient with metastatic bladder cancer. The patient was treated with everolimus, a drug that inhibits mTOR (mammalian target of rapamycin) signaling pathway. The results indicated the viability of using biomarkers to determine the probably response to certain medical treatments.

Michael suggested I look into HER/2neu, for which there is a clinical trial combining Il-2 with Herceptin; NY ESO-1, for which there is a vaccine; and VEGF and PDGF, which could lead to targeted drugs. PD-1 and PD-L1 have also been mentioned.

He also recommended that I contact Caris Life Sciences for information about their genetic testing and individualized cancer treatments. What I found out is there are a lot of questions to ask before you invest in genetic testing. This list apparently comes from Dr. Garrett Smith, MD, San Francisco.

Should I have biomarker analysis with molecular profiling?

♣ How effective and useful do you feel biomarker testing and analysis are?

♣ Is molecular profiling right for my cancer?

♣ What biomarkers are generally associated with my cancer?

♣ What could molecular profiling or biomarker analysis say about my cancer?

If molecular profiling is right for me, what do I need to know?

♣ What tests will I need to get? Will I need another biopsy or biopsies to have molecular profiling?

♣ Who will perform my biomarker analysis?

♣ How long will it take to get the results back?

What might molecular profiling reveal about my cancer?

♣ How will you use the results of my biomarker analysis?

♣ How likely is it that I will find a targeted treatment?

♣ What will happen if molecular profiling identifies an "off-label" or "off-compendium" treatment that might be effective for me?

What potential obstacles to this kind of testing do you see for me?

♣ Will insurance cover my biomarker testing and analysis? What about those treatments potentially recommended by that analysis?

♣ If my insurance or the cancer treatment center where I've been getting treatment don't support molecular profiling, what options do I have?

MEDICAL MARIJUANA

There has been a lot of talk and a lot of conflict about the benefits of medical marijuana for treatment of illnesses such as cancer. It has been proven to be helpful in treating a variety of symptoms for various medical conditions.

I have tried two forms of medical marijuana in 2014. The marijuana treatments were recommended by Michael Broffman and I was able to obtain the necessary documentation to use it.

The first time I took medical marijuana was in the form known as AC/DC during chemotherapy. He recommended me to take the tincture format. I began with a few drops and built up to 20 drops twice a day. I think this had a valuable effect.

The AC/DC formulation is composed of four parts CBD to one part THC. CBD is a cannabidiol, and THC is the substance that makes you high.

The second recommendation was to take medical marijuana in the form of CBD alone. This was in the form of capsules which I took daily. I didn't notice as big an effect as with AC/DC.

There are other strains and forms of medical marijuana and I recommend that you investigate which one is right for you.

DR. DEAN ORNISH'S SPECTRUM PROGRAM

Can lifestyle changes that affect your diet, stress response, exercise, and support have the effect of reducing or eliminating early stage prostate cancer and other kinds of illnesses?

Dr. Dean Ornish, MD, thinks so. In fact, he has proven his program to be workable under the strict requirements of a comprehensive randomized clinical trial.

Dr. Ornish's original research was with heart disease. He found that patients with heart disease who remained in the program for five years had significantly fewer cardiac events than the people in the control group.

I met Dean Ornish at the Academy for Guided Imagery (founded by Marty Rossman) conference in Hawaii in 1991. I was really impressed with his presentation and wanted to meet him. Marty introduced us and a few months later we played tennis together.

Dean Ornish's Spectrum method incorporates the four elements of what you eat, how much activity you have, how you manage stress, and how much love and support you have. Each of these elements corresponds to one of the *Seven Principles of Mindfulness in Healing* and you will recognize them as you come across them in your reading.

SUPPRESSED CANCER TREATMENTS

In my investigation of cancer treatments, I have found many modalities that have been suppressed by the FDA and big pharmaceutical companies. They have been suppressed because they did not pass the test of adding to the bottom line of the pharmaceutical companies or the pockets of the FDA.

One thing they have in common is that each one has added some value and life extension to people who have tried them out.

All of them have run into trouble with the FDA, AMA or big pharmaceutical companies.

These cures fall into three categories, according to Michael Broffman:

1. Low tech interventions – food, herbs, nutrition, acupuncture, etc.
2. Off-label non-standard intervention – FDA approved medications that can help you (see above)
3. Immunotherapy

I investigated cures in all three of these areas and decided on one as a fallback measure (GcMAF), but never followed up.

Most of these suppressed cancer treatments were presented in the documentary, *Cancer – The Forbidden Cures*[5]. The common denominator of all of these treatments is harassment by the United States Government, the FDA, and big pharmaceutical companies. It's no wonder that clinical trials, when attempted, had failed and that some of them are forbidden in the United States.

The Burzynski Clinic

Dr. Stanislaw Burzynski, MD, PhD is a Polish immigrant who obtained his Ph. D. in biochemistry from the Medical Academy in Lublin. His research involved the study of a group of peptides in people's urine.

He found that there were certain peptides in people that were free of cancer that were not present in people with cancer. He theorized that these peptides and peptide derivatives could be extracted from healthy people and given to sick people to cure cancer. He called them *antineoplastons*.

He founded his clinic in Houston, Texas in 1976, began manufacturing the antineoplastons, and treating cancer patients. He has had remarkable success with certain types of brain tumors and some success with other cancers. In fact, his success with these forms of brain cancer is better by far than any that modern medicine can claim. Why they continue to try to shut him down is truly a mystery to me.

I wrote to the clinic when I began research during the 2013 episode. I got a quick response with all kinds of forms to fill out and an extremely high price. I wrote back for them to give me specific details of what success they have had with treating bladder cancer and never got a response back.

Knowing the problems he had with big pharmaceutical companies, the FDA, and the Texas Medical Board, I wrote this method off, even though initially I thought it looked very promising.

Gerson Therapy

Gerson Therapy was founded by Dr. Max Gerson MD, a German-born American physician. The method he advocated was to adopt a plant-based diet, drink raw fruit and vegetable juices, take natural supplements, and utilize coffee enemas.

Max Gerson's philosophy is that natural treatments activate the body's own extraordinary ability to heal itself, just like my insight that "Healthy cells grow all by themselves."

This is another therapy that I seriously considered trying. I put it on hold because the clinic is in Mexico and the treatment is also rather expensive. The FDA, big pharmaceuticals, and the United States Government put a stop to the use of Gerson Therapy in the United States. Phooey! I think it has great promise.

If you look closely at some of the websites of the practitioners in *The Search for the Cures Continues*.[6], you are likely to find someone using parts or all of the Gerson therapy without calling it so.

Essiac

Essiac is an herbal concoction created by Rene Caisse that has worked for many people. It is not available in the United States, but it is available in Canada.

Essiac consists of four main herbs that grow in the wilderness of Ontario, Canada. They are burdock root, slippery elm inner bark, sheep sorrel and Indian rhubarb root.

I have not tried this remedy, but I certainly would not overlook the possibility of ordering it.

Hoxsey Formula

This treatment is another herbal formula discovered by Harry Hoxsey. It is used to cure some forms of cancer.

As usual, the FDA states, "There is no scientific evidence that it has any value to treat cancer, yet consumers can go online right now and find all sorts of false claims that Hoxsey treatment is effective against the disease."

This method uses a caustic herbal paste for skin cancers or a mixture of herbs for internal cancers. It is combined with laxatives, douches, vitamin supplements, and diet changes.

The combination of herbs was discovered when a horse with a tumor on its leg cured itself by grazing on wild plants growing in a meadow.

When I watched the video, I felt that this cure could possibly have some value, but I don't think I'd look further into this one. It is available online and at the Bio-Medical Center in Tijuana, Mexico.

Vitamin C

Everyone knows that the distinguished scientist, Dr. Linus Pauling, PhD proposed that vitamin C is a cure all for anything that ails you. Recently, I've learned that several of my close friends have been taking injections of massive doses of vitamin C. A couple of these friends either have cancer or have had cancer. They report an immediate boost in energy after treatment, and they go for treatments either once a week or once a month.

I considered doing intravenous treatments of vitamin C to support my immune system in response to the BCG treatments. I had an acupuncturist who was willing to prescribe it. When I emailed Michael Broffman about this, his response was that I could do it if I want but why not wait to see how the BCG works.

So far, there is no evidence that vitamin C can cure cancer. However, I do believe that it can boost the effectiveness of other cancer treatments (like BCG, for example).

Other Suppressed Cures

There are a number of other suppressed cures that you might want to investigate in extreme circumstances. You probably have heard of some of these. I'm just going to list them without any details.

- The New German Medicine proposed by Dr. Ryke Geerd Hamer
- Laetrile – vitamin B-17
- Shark cartilage
- Mistletoe (viscum album) – used by Rudolf Steiner and Suzanne Somers

- The Fungal Hypothesis proposed by Dr. Tullio Simoncini

They are time consuming, possibly expensive, and can cause reactions.

5 MAKE HEALTH-PROMOTING LIFESTYLE CHANGES

From my point of view, a supplement is something that you take internally or externally to help you feel better, correct a condition, or enhance your immune system. Supplements include, but are not limited to, vitamins, minerals, proteins, enzymes, herbs (including certain herbal teas), probiotics, and the like.

I've probably been taking supplements since I was a child. I remember my mother giving me cod liver oil, which was supposed to increase my omega 3 fatty acids (EPA and DHA) and provide vitamin A and D. It was yucky!

Only a trained physician, nutritionist, acupuncturist specializing in Chinese herbs, naturopath, chiropractor, and similar professionals are qualified to recommend supplements. Be wary of TV commercials, brochures you get in the mail and online ads because they can be harmful to your system or be counter indications of medicine and supplements that you are already taking.

My purpose here is not to recommend any supplements or lifestyle changes, but to report on what has worked for me. Many of the details of the exact supplements I took are not important.

The important thing is that supplements and lifestyle changes can be a factor in achieving overall better health and fitness. They can trigger your body's own resources for healing in surprising ways. Lifestyle changes, specifically, can activate your innate ability to heal yourself.

EXERCISE

I'm sure you know that exercise is good for you. But there are times during the healing process when you cannot possibly think of exercise. It is at these times that it is important to maintain your intention to exercise. Walking, even 30 minutes a day can help reduce inflammation.

During the course of my treatment for the first episode of bladder cancer, I was able to manage a little tennis once in a while. On other days, I needed some form of exercise that was less taxing to my system.

Strengthening Your Immune System Through Mind and Movement

For this purpose, I learned a series of exercises from a video tape called Strengthening Your Immune System through Mind and Movement[7] by Shirley Dockstader, MA, Marghe Mills, MED, and Dr. Richard Shames, MD, which can be ordered from the Pine Street Clinic. These were very healing when I did not have the strength to play tennis or do anything strenuous.

It begins with a posture called, *Standing Home*, from which all other movements begin and end. This is a basic posture in which your feet stand firmly on the ground, with your toes digging into the earth. Knees are soft, shoulders soft and dropped. Head floats, with chin and eyes level with the horizon.

Scan your body with your mind to release all tension. Count down from ten to settle your awareness somewhere in the very center of your body.

The movements are very easy to do and you will find comfort and confidence in doing them.

Mindful Movements

Another set of movements I found very useful were the *Mindful Movements*[8], created by Zen Master Thich Nhat Hanh (Thay), himself and the monks and nuns of Plum Village. Thay says, "When you calm your body and your emotions, you restore yourself, and you restore peace to the world around you."

I found these movements to be slightly more strenuous than the previous set, yet I was still able to do them fairly easily.

Thay guides you through a series of gentle exercises created specifically to cultivate a joyful awareness of the body and breath. These are the same "meditations in motion" that the monks and nuns of Plum Village Monastery use daily as a complement to their sitting meditation and walking meditation practices.

Arica Gym

The Arica Gym is the name that I learned for the Arica Psychocalisthenics program taught by Oscar Ichazo in his forty-day intensive training program. I learned the sequence of 23 movement and breathing exercises from my Fischer-Hoffman (now the Hoffman Process[9]) coach around 1974. I had previously been exposed to them in 1971, but they solidified in my life in '74.

For the past many years, I have been doing this set of exercises at least three times a week. I have added a set of restorative yoga practices and some Qi Gong exercises I learned from a good friend of mine who is also a master of Tai Chi.

This combination of exercises suits me to at tee. They activate the flow of vital energy through all the muscles, glands, organs, and tissues. The difficulty level varies from simple to "How in the hell am I going to be able to do that?"

You can benefit from these exercises if you are inclined to more physical activity than is required for the strengthening the immune system and mindful movements mentioned above. They virtually incorporate in different ways these two sets of exercise.

Tai Chi and Qi Gong

Tai Chi and Qi Gong are ancient Chinese martial arts, meditation, and exercise programs that can really help you on your healing journey. Classes in these two martial arts are all over.

A friend has tried to teach me some of the simpler movements of both of these. He was successful in getting some of the ideas across and some of them are part of my exercise regime about three times a week.

Medical research has shown that Tai Chi improves balance and general psychological heath, especially in older people. Qi Gong, on the other hand, has been the subject of research with regard to reliving hypertension and pain, without substantial conclusions. Scientists, especially in big pharmaceutical companies and the AMA, apparently don't approve of centuries of anecdotal evidence of the benefits of these practices.

THE CANCER DIET

If you read nothing else in this book, please pay close attention to and remember this: **cancer feeds on sugar**. Cancer feeds on false sugar. Therefore, first and foremost, eliminate sugar and other high glycemic index foods from your diet altogether.

Probably the most outrageous offender of human health is the soft drink industry. Whether you drink a diet cola or a regular cola, you are subject to feeding cancer cells in your body.

Diet drinks are especially bad. They indicate to the brain that some sugar is coming. When the real sugar fails to arrive, the brain sends out signals to crave more of what just got there. It wants you to have another diet drink.

Diet drinks usually contain an artificial sweetener called aspartame. This is particularly damaging to cells because it changes the amino acid ratio in your blood. There are 92 common side effects of aspartame!

The anticancer diet, says David Servan-Schreiber, M D, Ph D in his book, *Anticancer: a New Way of Life*[10], p. 4, Anticancer Action section,

> *"...is made up primarily of vegetables and legumes prepared with olive, canola, or flaxseed oil, or omega-3 butter, herbs, and spices. Unlike the traditional Western diet, meat and eggs are much less prominent; they are served as accompaniments in small amounts."*

According to Servan-Schreiber, the anticancer plate consists of vegetables, fruits, and vegetable proteins including lentils, peas, beans, tofu, etc.; herbs and spices, mainly turmeric, mint, thyme, rosemary and garlic; fats of olive, canola, or flaxseed oil, and omega-3 butter; grains in multigrain bread, whole-grain rice, quinoa, and bulgur; and optional animal proteins from fresh, organic free-range meats, omega-3 eggs, and organic free-range dairy products.

During the early stages of my 2013 episode of bladder cancer, my diet was restricted on the recommendation of Michael Broffman. The foods I was to avoid at that time were avocado, eggplant, soy, vinegar, pineapple, alcohol, chocolate, and wheat. I never got a full explanation of why this was so, but I was told that in general, these foods contradicted the workings of the Chinese herbs and supplements that he had me take.

I did quite well on this restriction. I even surprised myself at how little chocolate I had during this period. I could see and smell a whole plate of Mala's chocolate chip cookies without having a single one. I found gluten free bread to be less than optimum, but kept on it to avoid the wheat.

I made my own restriction of avoiding sugar because of a video I saw about the effects of sugar on the immune system and the knowledge that cancer feeds on sugar. For more information, please watch the documentary, *Hungry for Change*[11].

STRAWBERRIES, BLUEBERRIES, AND RASPBERRIES

Strawberries, blueberries, and raspberries are some of my all-time favorite foods. What they have in common is that they are rich in ellagic acid. Ellagic acid is a phytochemical that inhibits the genesis of tumors. They contain other phytochemicals called anthocyanins, which gives rise to their colors.

They also contain high amounts of vitamin C, which activates the immune system. For example, one cup of strawberries has more vitamin C than an orange. In addition, strawberries have two types of fiber that are wonderful for digestion. One type is tiny fibers in the meat of the fruit which connect the seeds to the core of the strawberry. The other type is found in the seeds, themselves.

Berries also contain significant amounts of antioxidants. Antioxidants supply electrons to reduce the inflammatory ability of free radicals.

NON-GMO FOODS

We are in deep trouble with our food system. This puts us in deep trouble with our health and our medical systems. This means that big pharmaceutical companies make billions of dollars and doctors and hospitals make lots of money because we are so sick. We are sick with cancer. We are sick with obesity. We are sick with diabetes. We are sick with heart disease.

All of these illnesses can be traced back to what we eat and environmental factors.

The food we eat now is mostly processed food. Why? Because it makes more money for big agricultural cartels (frankenfood companies[12]) and big brother chemical companies like Monsanto. They spend billions of dollars to convince us, our children and our grandchildren that they are good for us. They make us addicted to the sugar content in the processed foods, and you now know that cancer feeds on sugar.

The main reasons we are in trouble are GMO (genetically modified organisms) foods, too much sugar in just about all processed foods, which are, addicting, and the environmental factors of herbicides, pesticides and more.

In one documentary film that I saw, the filmmakers told the story of the devastating effects of GMO foods on a herd of cattle. These animals were allowed to glean the cotton fields somewhere in Norther India. For generations, they were safe from harm when they completed gleaning.

After the field had been planted with GMO cotton, the herd was again allowed to glean the fields after harvest. All of the animals perished. What do you think happened to them? Could the same be happening to us when we consume GMO foods?

Here are four steps that you can do right now:
1. Cut out refined and artificial sugars from your diet.
2. Stop buying GMO and processed foods and the frankenfood companies will have to stop making them. For example, boycott Cheerios and donuts.
3. Shop at farmer's markets when possible and buy organic fruits and vegetables as much as possible.
4. When you eat meat, be sure it is from free range animals and prefer organic.

MINDFUL CONSUMPTION

One of the principle causes of unrest in our society is the constant desire for more material objects. Shopping seems to be our national pastime. We continually want more and aren't satisfied with what we have.

The problem is not in the buying of shiny objects. The problem is in our craving for them. We crave the sensation of owning these new, shiny objects. It is this sensation that we really want and desire and not necessarily the objects themselves.

Sometimes we buy things to cover up our loneliness, anxiety, and other suffering. This is especially true when we reach into the refrigerator, even when we are not hungry.

Mindful consumption means to recognize that the cravings we have will only lead to more cravings, more desire, more clinging, and more suffering. When we are trying to change our lifestyle, mindful consumption is a good practice to observe.

Mindful consumption develops from our awareness of ourselves and our connections with our ancestors, descendants, and our society. When we practice mindful consumption we acknowledge the causes and conditions that bring our basic needs to us. We realize all the hard work that farmers do to plant, harvest, and deliver food to our tables. We are grateful for their efforts.

Thich Nhat Hanh says, "Mindful consumption is the way to heal ourselves and the world." Mindful consumption is a way for us to restore our connection and balance with the natural world. This way, we can contribute to sustaining our environment and making the earth a safer place for our children and our children's children.

Here are some ideas on what you can do to consume mindfully. First of all we need to cultivate good health, both physical and mental, for ourselves, our families and our society. Without this, there will be nothing left for future generations.

Another thing we can do is to turn off our televisions, especially commercial television. Do you know how harmful some of the drugs they advertise are for us and our society? Turning off the news and commercials can give you a sense of peace that you can cultivate each day.

Spending less time on the internet is also a good idea. Certain web sites have the property of encouraging mindless consumption and they make it very easy for us to acquire shiny objects.

If we take shorter showers, buy locally produced fruits and vegetables, eat more vegetarian meals, and avoid plastic containers, we will contribute to a cleaner environment. Recycling paper, plastics, and aluminum will also help.

Did you know that the amount of water it takes to raise one pound of beef for consumption by humans is equivalent to all the water you use in a year of daily showers? This is really a wake-up call for us to minimize our meat consumption to the levels suggested by Servan-Schreiber.

My introduction to mindful consumption came more than thirty years ago when I heard Thich Nhat Hanh say, "If the West stops drinking alcohol by fifty percent, we could feed the whole world."

I took this as a sign to not consume alcohol and become aware of how I was consuming. I haven't had alcohol since that time and I am reluctant to buy anything that I don't absolutely need. Instead of buying books, I rent them from the library.

6 PRACTICE DAILY MEDITATION

The seven principles of mindfulness in healing would not be complete without a chapter on daily meditation practices. I have to say, that in my experience, my daily practice provided me with the tools I needed to achieve a remission from muscle invasive bladder cancer twice in the past nineteen years.

Mindfulness was the cornerstone of all of the other principles that you have read about so far. This one may be the most important one for changing the direction of your life.

I made this into a separate chapter because mindfulness meditation can and should be practiced on a daily basis, whether or not you are dealing with a health crisis. The chapters on alternatives and supplements as well as the other principles can be carried on into your daily life as well, but their main focus is healing.

If you are beginning a daily physical exercise program, you don't begin by lifting 500 pounds. You build up to it gradually.

Just like physical exercise, mental exercise or meditation is begun at an easy level that even three- or four-year-old children can do. You begin practicing meditation for as little as nine minutes a day and work your way up to longer periods. In addition, as you continue to practice, you will notice that you are able to return to your meditation experience from distractions more and more quickly.

Benefits of Mindfulness Meditation

Mindfulness meditation helps you begin to experience peace within you and around you. Peace may not come all at once, but if you practice for at least nine minutes a day for three weeks in a row without missing a day I bet you will find more peace in your life.

Next, you may experience your heart opening to the people you love and who love you and begin to enjoy the wonders of life around you.

You may see more clearly how the earth we live on is really a wonderful place to be. You probably will find more enjoyment in flowers, birds, trees, animals, and other life forms, recognizing that they too want happiness and to avoid suffering.

Your own feelings about yourself may reach a point where you are happy most of the day. You may experience a glimpse of the beauty and radiance of your own true nature.

You may be able to answer such questions as, "Who am I", or "What is my purpose in life?" In any case, the increased knowledge of your inner self will inspire you to keep on practicing for many years to come.

Many practitioners find that their health improves drastically as stress is reduced or eliminated from their lives. In my way of thinking, stress is the extra suffering we put on ourselves over and above the challenges that life brings. Mindfulness is the path to lessening the hold of the stress of our addictions and brings about increased wellness.

Quite often, mindfulness practitioners experience a degree of happiness far above their normal state. This happiness comes from the freedom experienced during sitting quietly and recognizing that one can be content with one's own life situation just as it is. This freedom provides an insight into taking life in the present moment, without putting anything extra on it in the way of stress or extra effort to get things accomplished.

Life seems to be experienced "in the now" – not just on the tennis court, but also in playing, exercising, working, creating, loving, eating, sleeping, dreaming, and other aspects of the whole wondrous experience of living.

As you continue to practice, you may find that your addictions have less hold on your mind. Suppose you feel addicted to caffeine in one form or another, e. g., Starbucks or Peet's coffee, chocolate, TV shows, and the like. In the past, you would not stop a moment to think about getting that extra cup of coffee or having that additional piece of chocolate or watching that TV show.

However, with mindfulness practice, you start to become aware of these kinds of urges as seeds before they reach the level of mind consciousness causing you to act impulsively. You then notice, "My little coffee addiction – I know you are there and I am here for you. Please remain a seed for a little while longer and I will take care of you."

A benefit that people experience out the gate is that of relaxation. Mindfulness practice brings on the relaxation response in most people, even the very first time they try meditation. The feeling of relaxation that comes with sitting silently can make you feel like you have slept peacefully for some length of time. You may come out of your session being quite refreshed and ready to take on your abundant life.

Another benefit that sitting quietly brings is the possibility of insight into various aspects of your life. Insight is the process of recognizing something important in just about any phase of existence. As you practice, sensations arise that give you a new understanding of your life situation.

Long time practitioners begin to notice a fondness and reverence for life. Aware of the suffering caused by the destruction of life, they commit themselves to cultivating compassion and finding ways to protect the lives of people, animals, plants and minerals.

They also try to minimize the amount of killing in the world and are themselves dedicated not to kill, even be it a tiny spider, or to let others kill.

Also, long-time practitioners become aware of the challenges caused by exploitation, social injustice, stealing, and oppression, and they commit themselves to practicing generosity by sharing their time, energy, and material resources with those in need.

They cultivate loving kindness and compassion for all beings and respect their rights and property. Along the same lines, experienced practitioners regard the sanctity of sexual conduct of prime importance and experience sexual relationship in situations when there is love and a long-term commitment. They do everything possible to protect children from sexual abuse and try to keep couples and families together.

Experienced practitioners cultivate deep listening and loving speech. They listen with full attention and try not to judge what they hear. They speak their truth as much as possible in order to help resolve conflicts and protect their families and communities from harm.

Furthermore, experienced practitioners are mindful in what they consume. They avoid alcohol and other intoxicants and ensure their well-being by eating properly and not over-spending.

They work to transform violence, fear, anger, and confusion in themselves and in their environment.

There are several attitudes adopted by mindfulness practitioners that trigger skillful behavior when it comes to life situations. These qualities of the heart, as they are known, include generosity, morality, patience, and determination, among others. These qualities provide incentives for mindfulness in daily life.

TYPES OF MEDITATION

If you examine the religious traditions around the world, you will find that each one has its own types of meditation practices. From the ecstatic dance of Amazonian shamans to the quiet sitting meditation of Zen monks in Japan, you will find everything in between.

It is safe to say that all forms of meditation have more or less the common goal of living a better life; and developing compassion and wisdom. Some forms have even more lofty goals.

There are a great many good books, YouTube videos, and magazines about meditation. To do the subject justice would take a couple of volumes by itself. So in this section you will learn a few different types of meditation that can help you feel better, heal, and start on the path to well-being with a daily mindfulness practice.

Please try each one of these until you get the feel of it and then chose one or more for your daily practice. Perhaps a story from the time of the Buddha will inspire you to begin.

The Buddha was staying at his meditation center in Savatthi in Northern India. One young man would come to listen to Buddha's evening discourses on a regular basis.

One time, he came a little bit early and found the Buddha alone. He asked the Buddha why, with all his power and compassion, he doesn't liberate all of his followers.

The Buddha answered his question with another question, something he was prone to do. Noticing that the young man was not from Savatthi, he asked him where he was from.

The young man replied that he was from a town called Rajagaha, quite a ways away from where the Buddha was staying.

The conversation continues with the Buddha asking him about whether he goes to Rajagaha, why he goes there, and so on.

Ultimately, we find out that the path from Savatthi to Rajagaha is well-known and the young man would be willing to reveal that path to any interested party. The Buddha directs the conversation so that the young man realizes that unless the people follow the path from Savatthi to Rajagaha, they will never get there.

Similarly, the young man, or anyone else who knows about the Buddha's path to awakening, will never get there if they don't follow the path themselves.

The Buddha never claimed to be anything else but a normal person who found the way. He never claimed to be a god or angel or anything other than a human being. When asked what was different about him, he would reply, "I am awake," which is the meaning of Buddha.

In the sections that follow, you will be introduced to what are considered to be the most fundamental meditation practices for beginners. If you are not a beginner, you probably will learn something from following the instructions that follow the descriptions of the practices.

MINDFULNESS OF BREATHING

Speaking of the Buddha, the first meditation practice he ever taught was mindfulness of breathing. What is mindfulness of breathing?

It is actually quite simple but not easy. To be mindful of breathing you have to know when you are breathing in. You have to know when you are breathing out. You have to recognize a long breath as a long breath and you have to recognize a short breath as a short breath.

To practice mindfulness of breathing, find a comfortable position where you will not be disturbed for nine short minutes. This could be a cushion on the floor where you would sit with your back straight. You could also do the practice sitting in a comfortable chair or lying down in your bed or on the floor.

After a few weeks of practice of nine-minute meditation, you can gradually begin to increase the length to twenty, thirty, or forty-five minutes, or whatever length is comfortable for you.

I chose nine minutes because it is fairly short and you should be able to find nine minutes sometime during your busy day. If you wish, you can set a timer on your cell phone or other device. Although this is preferred at the beginning, you can do without it, especially if you are taking your nine-minute meditation break on a bus, ferry, or train on your way to work.

If you would prefer to be guided in this practice, please visit the "First Mindfulness Meditation Practice[13]" on the **Meditation Practices[4]** web site right under the "Mindfulness" menu item. There are five other guided meditations there, as well. You can listen to them on your smartphone or tablet using your web browser. Ear phones are recommended.

The Practice of Mindfulness of Breathing

Step 1: Once you are seated or lying down, close your eyes and take a minimum of three, deep belly breaths. Breath in all the way to the bottom of your diaphragm and breath out at the approximately the same rate.

Step 2: Next withdraw yourself into yourself and become aware of your meditation position. Become aware of your body. Feel where your body contacts the cushion, chair, or bed. Spend a few moments noticing how you feel doing this part of the process.

Step 3: Be aware of no other spaces than the spaces that you occupy. Be aware of no other times but this time. Be here, be now. Be here now.

Step 4: Now as your breathing becomes normal, begin to follow your breathing with your mind. Breathing in, know that you are breathing in. Breathing out, know that you are breathing out.

You may feel your breath mostly in your abdomen, chest, throat, windpipe, or nostrils. You can chose whichever place you want to focus on, as long as it feels natural to you.

To help you out at the beginning, it is possible to use the following device to increase your ability to concentrate. When you breathe in, say to yourself, "I know I am breathing in," or even more simply, "In." When you breathe out, say to yourself, "I know I am breathing out," or more simply, "Out."

You can actually choose your own set of word triggers, based on your experience. For example, once I recited the little poem at the beginning of Chapter 1, I used "Healthy" on the in breath and "Free" on the outbreath.

If you experience your breath deeply in your abdomen, you can use a very old technique of repeating "Rising" when you breathe in and "Falling" when you breathe out.

In Zen practice, they teach counting the inhalations or the exhalations from one to ten, repeatedly. If you use this technique and lose the count, simply begin again.

Speaking of losing the count, there undoubtedly will be times when your mind is flooded with "should's" and "have to's" and you are distracted from your breathing. When this happens, simply bring your mind back to your breathing and place whatever crossed your mind into the back of your mind to be attended to later. Let these kinds of thoughts go as if they were white clouds drifting across the clear blue sky.

Distractions happen frequently, even in the most experienced meditators. They have learned to let them go and return to their object of meditation, in this case, their breathing in and out, without further ado.

Don't let it worry you or give you the feeling of failure if you session is full of thoughts and distractions. Consider them part of your learning process

Step 5: When the bell on your timer rings, or you learn that your nine-minute meditation period is over, slowly open your eyes and return to your normal daily activities. It may be a good idea to write down any thoughts or insights that you have experienced during your meditation session. Keeping a diary of this sort can be very beneficial.

Please remember that it is more important to meditate than to worry about improving your meditation skills. Consistency is more important than technique when you are first beginning to meditate.

For more details, and for guided meditation practices of this type of meditation, please visit the **Meditation Practices**[4] website and visit each of the mindfulness meditation practices under the menu, "*Mindfulness*," just below the banner.

For a detailed online meditation course, try **9 Minute Meditation**[14], where you will learn more than a dozen different meditation practices to try out at your own pace. Not all of the information is available when you sign up. Lessons are made available at the rate of three or four a week.

Variations – Pebble Meditation

You will be happy to learn that Zen Master Thich Nhat Hanh teaches children from about age three how to do pebble meditation. He first has the children gather four lovely stones and put them in a pouch for safe keeping.

When they are ready to do pebble meditation, they place their pouches on their left and take a few relaxing deep breaths. Then they remove the first pebble and place it in their right hands.

The first pebble represents a flower. The children are taught to say to themselves while they are breathing in, "I see myself as a flower." They are taught to say to themselves while they are breathing out, "I feel fresh." More advance students, can simply say, "Flower" when they breathe in and "Fresh" when they breathe out.

The children are taught that they are a flower in the garden of humanity and that when they are dwelling in the present moment, they are always fresh.

They close their right hand on the pebble and close their eyes. They carry this on for several breaths – maybe ten to twenty or so, or as few as four or six.

Then they put the flower pebble on the right, reach into the pouch, pull out the second pebble and place it in their right hand. The second pebble represents a mountain. The mountain represents the quality of solidity inside of them.

This time, while they hold the pebble in their right hand, they are taught to say to themselves when they breathe in, "I see myself as a mountain." When they breathe out they are taught to say to themselves, "I feel solid as a mountain." Advanced students use the words "Mountain," and "Solid."

They are taught that when they feel solid as a mountain, nothing can knock them over. They feel very stable.

They put the pebble from their right hand down next to them and pick up the third pebble.

The next pebble represents a pond or lake of clear water. When the pond or lake is completely still, it will reflect the mountains in the distance, the nearby trees, and flowers on the shore. It will reflect things just as they are. They are taught that the water reflecting represents what is real, what is true. When their minds are calm, they can see things clearly.

They pick up the third pebble, place in right hand, and repeat these phrases when the breath in, "I feel I am water." Breathing out, they say, "I reflect things as they are." More advance students use, "Water" and "Reflecting."

They put the water pebble down and pick up the fourth pebble.

This pebble represents space, and space represents freedom.

The children are taught that when they are free, they are truly happy. They have everything they need to be happy in the present moment.

The words for this pebble are "I see myself as space" while breathing in and "I feel free" while breathing out. Or simply, "Space," "Free."

Now comes the point of this whole meditation practice.

The children are ready to pick up the pebbles and place them back in the pouch. They will carry the pouch with them as much as possible.

When they feel angry or irritated, they can reach into the pouch and pick up the flower pebble. They can touch the freshness that that flower pebble represents and calm their anger. They can become fresh again themselves.

When they feel frightened or uneasy, they can reach into the pouch and pick up the mountain pebble. This will give them a feeling of solidity. The feeling of being solid will counteract their fear or uneasiness.

If their mind is not clear and they have a lot of emotions coming up, they can pick up the water pebble and begin to see things more clearly. Their minds can become calm and they can reflect things, just as they are.

When they are feeling a little hemmed in, trapped, or otherwise uncomfortable, they can pick up the space pebble and touch real freedom. The can recognize that they are free just as they are. This will reduce their feelings of being uncomfortable.

If you want to watch a video or two describing the pebble meditation, please visit the **Meditation Practices**[4] website and search for "pebble meditation."

WALKING MEDITATION

Before and during the time of the Buddha, monks and nuns would walk slowly from their hermitage to the village to beg for food. Their minds would be fully attentive to each step they took.

When they reached the village, they would go from door to door with their begging bowls. They would knock on the doors of the villagers and wait patiently for them to respond.

When the door was opened, they would bow in deep respect and place their bowl in easy reach of the villages. They would accept with gratitude any food offerings they would receive.

When their bowls were full, they would walk slowly back to their hermitage and, say a few prayers of thanksgiving for the food they received and eat each morsel in total mindfulness. This is called mindfulness of eating, which we will cover later.

In the time of the Buddha, the members of his community would only eat twice a day, and nothing after noon. This gave them the time they needed for meditation and to do their daily chores.

During the war in Vietnam, there was a poignant moment in the demilitarized zone. There was continuous gun fire across this zone. A group of monks in orange robes started walking across the middle of the zone. Both sides of the war stopped their gunfire as the monks walked across. They were all safe.

This shows you the power of walking meditation. The participants are walking not only for themselves, but for the benefit of the people around them. They demonstrated the power of a moment of peace.

Walking meditation is one of the most important activities for someone with a life-threatening or milder condition. For me, it became indispensable.

Since I wasn't able to play tennis as frequently as I would like to have, I relied on walking meditation to provide some form of movement as well as an opportunity to feel what it feels like to walk.

The difference between walking meditation and going for a walk is subtle. When you go for a walk, you must pay attention to where you are going, but your mind can go anywhere else.

With walking meditation, you must also pay attention to where you are going, but in this case, you are aware that you are walking with each step, moment by moment.

When you lift your right foot, you know you are lifting your right foot. When you place your right foot, you know that you are placing your right foot.

When you lift your left foot, you know you are lifting your left foot. When you place your left foot, you know that you are placing your left foot. Each step is done with total awareness.

A famous Zen proverb states, "In walking, just walk. In sitting, just sit. Above all, don't wobble." Of course, it is all right to wobble! Just wobble mindfully!

The Practice of Walking Meditation

There are basically two types of walking meditation. The first type is practiced indoors with a predetermined path, either in a circle or up and down a corridor. The physical environment usually determines whether you walk in a circle or up and down a corridor. You may even find yourself walking in a rectangle if there are obstructions that you need to walk around. This type of walking meditation is usually considerably slower than the next.

The other type of walking meditation is outside, where there are lots of choices. You may not necessarily choose a destination at the beginning of your walking meditation.

Both types of walking meditation have their benefits and advantages. Walking outdoors has the disadvantage of many distractions, but walking outdoors can be wonderful when you walk mindfully and learn to appreciate the wonders of life.

In an advanced form of walking meditation when you are walking outdoors, you may come across something that captures your attention like a beautiful flower, a friendly cat or dog, a beautiful sunset, beautiful ripples on a pond, creek, or river, a field of grasses that look totally amazing, or anything else. In this case, you can stop to appreciate these wonders of life and then continue on.

Step 1: Decide on when and where you want to do walking meditation. If you are indoors, you might want to plan a period of nine minutes of walking meditation in between two periods of sitting meditation. This is what is usually done in sitting groups, although the periods of sitting meditation are considerably longer.

If you are practicing outdoors away from your home, drive there comfortably and mindfully and begin your walking meditation the moment you get out of your car. The period can be any time between nine and thirty minutes or more. Be sure to walk mindfully from your car to the path for your meditation.

What does it mean to walk mindfully?

Step 2: When you walk mindfully, you are aware of each step. When you lift your left foot, you know you are lifting your left foot and all of your attention is on the lifting. When you place your left foot, all you attention is on placing your left foot.

When you lift your right foot, you are aware that you are lifting your right foot and all of your attention is on your right foot. When you are placing your right foot, all of your attention is on the placing.

To make matters easier, each time you lift either foot, you can say to yourself, "Lifting." When you place either foot, you can say to yourself, "Placing."

So you carry on like this, "Lifting... placing... lifting... placing." Or you can use any words that help you to focus on your lifting and placing of each foot.

In my personal experience, I learned to use my own poem that you read in the Introduction. When I lift my left foot, I say to myself, "Healthy." When I lift my right foot, I say to myself, "Free." I began this in 1997 and still practice it today.

Step 3: When the time period that you have allocated for walking meditation ends, please don't stop there. There is no reason to discontinue walking meditation even though the formal period of walking meditation is over!

Walk mindfully to the kitchen or wherever else you are going in your house if you are practicing indoors. Walk mindfully to your car if you are walking outdoors. Drive mindfully to your next destination.

After you have become used to this type of meditation practice, you might want to apply it to other aspects of your life. For example, when you wash the dishes, simply wash the dishes. Don't wash your worries, your cares, or your anxieties. Leave them behind.

When you fold the laundry, simply fold the laundry. Don't fold any of your anger, your fear, or your stress into the clothes. Just fold the clothes.

Do you get the idea? Bring mindfulness into everything that you do and you'll find that your life flows a lot easier.

For more information on walking meditation, please visit the **Meditation Practices**[4] website and search for "walking meditation." You will find many interesting articles for you to read and some entertaining videos for you to watch.

THE BODY SCAN AND DEEP RELAXATION

The body scan meditation is really two meditations in one, depending on how you use it. The first use is simply to scan the body from head to foot or from foot to head to feel the sensations you experience in each part of your body.

You will find that in some parts of your body, you will enjoy a pleasant sensation; while in other parts of your body, you will experience an unpleasant sensation. At some parts of your body, you will experience a neutral sensation, one that is neither pleasant nor unpleasant.

What you will discover when you do this form of meditation is that all the sensations are of the nature to change. They simply are impermanent. They come into being, stay for a while (maybe a long time), and eventually go away.

The second form of body scan is for the purpose of deep relaxation. You will visit each part of your body and invite each part to relax, let go, and release.

Do you remember the first type of meditation that the Buddha taught? Refer back to mindfulness of breathing if you don't. Well, the second type of meditation the Buddha taught is be aware of your body as described above, and release all the tensions in your body.

Deep Relaxation Meditation Practice

In this meditation practice, you will learn to put your attention on various parts of your body and encourage those parts to relax, let go, and release. You should read through this entire section before you practice it so that you get a better sense of what to do.

This deep relaxation meditation can be done sitting comfortably in a chair or on a cushion, or lying down. You might want to try lying down the first time you do it. This one can take a little longer than nine minutes, and it all depends on how long you spend relaxing the various parts of your body.

You may even want to practice this meditation when you are lying in your bed in preparation for deep, relaxing sleep. You can allow yourself to drift off to sleep if you want.

This meditation can be done from the top of your head to the bottom of your feet and toes or the other way around. It is totally a matter of personal preference whether you begin at the top of your head or at the bottom of your feet and toes.

Step 1: Begin with at least three deep breaths all the way down into your belly. Make sure that you can sense the rise and fall of your abdomen. Let the out breaths be shorter than the in breaths and let them be a real letting-go type of breath.

Step 2: When you are ready, bring your awareness to the top of your head. Feel the sense of how the top of the head feels. Invite the top of your head to relax, let go, and release.

Now repeat this process for your forehead, eyebrows, and your eyelids. Take as much time as you want. There is no need to rush.

Now invite your eyes to relax, let go, and release. Your eyes provide you with the ability to see the wonders of life. You might say to your eyes, "I am happy and grateful now that I have eyes in good condition to see the wonders of life." You can use any phrase that strikes your fancy or simply move on.

Next, relax your cheeks and nostrils. Since you nostrils are the main entry point for oxygen to come into your body, you might say to your nostrils and nose, "I am happy and grateful now that my nose is in good condition to smell the odors of life." Again, you can use any phrase that you want or no phrase at all. It is totally up to you.

Next, invite your lips to relax. You may feel them gently touch each other or you may not. In either case you know that your lips are extremely sensitive to touch and this sensation could remind you that you have tactile sensations all over your body. You might say to yourself, "I am happy and grateful now that my sense of touch is working normally and I can experience wonderful sensations when in contact with the world around me." You can use this phrase or any one of your own choosing or no phrase at all.

Move now inside your mouth and invite your tongue to relax. Your sense of taste resides partially in your tongue and partially in your nose. You may want to say to yourself, "I am happy and grateful now that I have a tongue in normal condition to experience the tastes of good fruits and vegetables. I am happy and grateful now that I can use my tongue, breath, and vocal cords to speak lovingly and offer my gifts to the world." Of course, you don't need to say anything at all or you can make up your own saying.

Invite your chin and jaws to relax, let go, and release.

Follow the line of your jaws to your ears and invite your ears to relax, let go, and release. You might say to your ears, "I am happy and grateful now that my ears are in good enough condition that I can listen deeply and respond to the cries of the world." Or, you can just move on to the next step.

Now it is time to invite your whole head and face to relax, let go, and release. Spend a few extra moments regarding your head and face before moving on to the next part.

Invite your neck to relax all the way around. Invite your neck to let go, and release. Invite it to relax from the inside out and from the outside in.

Relax your shoulders, upper arms and elbows, your forearms and wrists, your hands, fingers, and fingertips. Take your time moving down from your shoulders to your fingertips. This is the part of your body where you will most likely feel lively sensations. You may have never taken time to experience them before, but they are certainly there.

Moving back up, relax your fingers, hands, arms and shoulders. Take your time. There is nothing pressing right now.

Please bring your attention now to the place where the skull meets your spine. Invite the top of your spine down into the top of your back to relax, let go, release.

Moving gently down your spine and back, invite that part of your spine between your shoulder blades and the shoulder blades themselves to relax, let go, release.

Moving gently down your spine to the mid-section of your back, invite that part of your spine and your mid-back to gently relax, let go, release.

Moving gently down to the lower part of your spine including your sacrum, and your tailbone, and your lower back, invite those parts to relax, let go, release.

Now slowly move your attention back up your spine from the tail bone to the place where skull meets the spine and insure that every muscle and every nerve in your total back and spine has had an opportunity to relax, let go, and release.

Now feel the upper part of your torso – your chest, lungs, and heart. Take two slow deep abdominal breaths and invite these parts to relax deeply (if you are still awake)! Invite these parts to relax, let go, and release.

You may want to say to your lungs, "I am happy and grateful now that I have two lungs with which to breathe in and breathe out and provide the oxygen that my cells need to thrive." You may skip this phrase if you want.

Bring your attention to your heart. Do you feel it beating? You may now say to your heart, "I am happy and grateful now that my heart keeps on beating and bringing fresh oxygenated blood to my cells." You may also skip this if you want.

Continuing with your upper body, you might want to recognize your liver, gallbladder, spleen, esophagus, stomach, pancreas, kidneys, and adrenal glands and other glands and organs for all they do to keep you heathy and alive. After all, these are known as your "vital organs!"

Invite the muscles and nerves, in your abdomen to relax, let go, and release. Invite your intestines, bladder, and sex organs to do the same. Spend a little time with these other vital organs.

Now move into your pelvis and hips and invite them to relax, let go, and release.

Next, invite your thighs, knees, calves, ankles, heels, and toes to relax, let go and release. Do this part rather slowly. There is a lot of volume to cover.

Now you have relaxed all the muscles, nerves, organs, glands, and other vital parts of your body from your toes all the way up to the top of your head and from the top of your head to the tips of your toes. You should by now be completely and deeply relaxed.

Lie there for a while and feel the wonderful feeling of being totally relaxed. There is nothing to do. There is nowhere to go. Just be there and allow your whole body to relax, let go, and release.

When you are ready, if you haven't fallen asleep, take a couple of deep breaths, stretch your body and return to the rest of your day or evening.

The best time to do this deep relaxation is in the morning just after you wake up. The second best time to do it is in the evening before you go to bed. Then you can allow yourself to float of to a deep, relaxing sleep.

For more information about this type of meditation, please visit **Meditation Practices**[4] and search for *"relaxation."*

LOVING KINDNESS MEDITATION

When thousands of people were asked, "What do you want in a relationship," the vast majority said they want kindness – loving kindness.

I know very well what it feels like to receive true loving kindness. My wife, Mala, is an expert at giving it. You can see it in the way she treats our children. You can see it in the way she treats her many "best" friends. You can see it in the way she addresses strangers.

Loving kindness is one of the four "immeasurable minds" or "*Brahma Viharas*" – divine abodes or graces that the Buddha taught 2,600 years ago. A *vihara* is a dwelling place or divine abode in Sanskrit. These are the four elements of true love.

The word for loving kindness in Sanskrit is *maitri*, while in Pali, the language the Buddhist scriptures are written in, the word for loving kindness is *metta*. The reason I bring this up is that loving kindness meditation is often referred to as *metta* meditation.

The other divine abodes are compassion (*karuna* in both Pali and Sanskrit), sympathetic joy (*mudita* in both Pali and Sanskrit) and equanimity (*upeksha* in Sanskrit and *upekkha* in Pali). Zen Master Thich Nhat Hanh often speaks of inclusiveness as the fourth divine abode.

The teaching is that developing one of these graces is tied directly to developing them all. If you have loving kindness, it is possible to manifest compassion, sympathetic joy and equanimity. If you have sympathetic joy, you can manifest loving kindness, compassion and equanimity. And so forth.

They are called "immeasurable" because practicing them will bring you immeasurable happiness and eventually you will be able to embrace the whole world. People around you will notice your happiness and they will become happier also.

When I first began to practice these graces, I noticed that it was relatively easy for me to develop sympathetic joy, especially for and with my children. I would experience waves of joy and happiness when they reported good things that were happening in their lives.

I believe that one of the first times this occurred with the four immeasurable minds as a conscious practice was when one of my daughters was playing on her high school tennis team. I was filled with joy that she was participating in something I love.

It didn't take me long to connect the dots and begin to have a regular *metta* practice. Once this began, I realized that compassion and equanimity were just around the corner. And, they too, began to arise often in my life.

One time in 2009, I was invited to speak at my niece's wedding celebration in Israel. I proceeded to speak about how the newlyweds could enhance their love life by practicing the four immeasurable minds. They now have two young girls, which I am sure, give them many opportunities for loving kindness, happiness and sympathetic joy.

The Loving Kindness Meditation Practice

The scriptures tell us that for someone to develop loving kindness for others; they must first develop loving kindness for themselves. This may not be as easy as it seems, as several people told me of their difficulties with this.

These kinds of people have low self-esteem and need the benefits of a qualified teacher. However, if they begin with the first loving kindness meditation practice and stick with it persistently, eventually things will begin to clear up and they will begin to develop compassion, joy, and equanimity.

The traditional way of doing loving kindness meditation is to shower the loving kindness blessings (coming soon) on yourself. This is because people often have difficulty loving others if they can't love themselves. This may be continued on its own for several weeks or months until you feel really comfortable moving on.

This is usually followed by bringing to mind someone close to you. It could be your spouse, child, parent, grandparent, grandchild, or close friend. You'll see below that you can also pick a group, such as your immediate family members. Then you shower the loving kindness blessings on that person or group.

Following this, you choose someone you have difficulty with, whether it is a spouse, parent, grandparent, child, grandchild, friend, acquaintance or stranger. Then you shower the loving kindness blessings on that person.

Next, in the traditional method, you shower loving kindness

blessing on strangers, like the people who serve you in the grocery store or shopping center. Then proceed to shower loving kindness blessings of all sentient beings and planet Earth.

Like the traditional method, we begin by showing loving kindness blessings on ourselves.

Take a comfortable position sitting straight on a cushion or a straight-back chair. You can even do this meditation lying down, if necessary, but try not to fall asleep.

Step 1: Begin the practice by taking a minimum of three deep breaths. As you breathe in, follow your in breath all the way in. As you breathe out, follow your out breath all the way out.

Step 2: When you are ready, allow your breathing to become normal and withdraw yourself into yourself. Become aware of your meditation seat. Be aware of no other spaces but these spaces. Be aware of no other times but these times. Be here. Be now. Be here now.

Step 3: Now bring your attention to the place in your body where you feel most yourself. This could be your heart center or anywhere else that pleases you.

Shower these loving kindness blessings on yourself.

May I be safe from internal and external harm.
May I have a calm, clear mind and a peaceful, loving heart.
May I be physically strong, healthy and vital.
*May I experience love, joy, wonder and wisdom in this life, **just as it is**.*

Sit with each of these blessings for a while. Let them penetrate through the barriers of fear, uncertainty, and doubt. Let them bring a feeling of deep well-being into your heart-mind.

You are welcome to repeat them as many times as necessary to feel comfortable in yourself. I often repeat them three times.

Step 4: When you are ready, bring to mind the most important people in your life – your spouse, your children, your grandchildren, your parents, your grandparents, your significant other, or any others that you choose. You will have a chance later to bring to mind your siblings and their families and your closest friends.

When you have brought each person to mind that you want to at this time, shower these loving kindness blessings on them:

May you be safe from internal and external harm.
May you have a calm, clear mind and a peaceful, loving heart.
May you be physically strong, healthy and vital.
May you experience love, joy, wonder and wisdom in this life, **just as it is**.

Sit with each of these blessings for a while and let them spread out to the universe and reach your loved ones in a special way.

Step 5 (optional): When you are ready, call to mind your siblings, their families, and your truest friends.

Shower the above loving kindness blessings on this group of people that you also love with all your heart. Be sure to sit for a moment with any feelings that arise as you are doing this meditation.

Step 6: When you are ready, bring to mind people you know who are suffering from illness, disappointment, loss, despair, sadness, grief, fear, and so forth. You don't even have to know these people very well. They can even be people from the previous blessings. They can even be friends of friends or perfect strangers that you heard were experiencing a lot of difficulty. It is perfectly all right to include yourself in this group.

Bring each person in this group to your heart-mind and shower the above loving kindness blessings on them. Take your time and sit with each of these people as you recite the blessings.

Step 7 (optional): Now imagine our planet Earth, floating like a jewel in the vast emptiness of space. Picture the snow-capped mountains, the vast deserts, the green forests and croplands, and, of course, the blue oceans, rivers and lakes. Take you time to visualize sentient beings living in cities and in rural areas. Take you time to consider the animals that roam the forests and grasslands, and all the fish and life in the deep blue sea.

Now shower these loving kindness blessings on all sentient beings:

May we be safe from internal and external harm.
May we have a calm, clear mind and a peaceful, loving heart.
May we be physically strong, healthy and vital.
*May we experience love, joy, wonder and wisdom in this life, **just***
as it is.

Remember what Carl Sagan said,

The surface of the Earth is the shore of the cosmic ocean. On this
shore, we've learned most of what we know. Recently, we've waded
a little way out, maybe ankle-deep, and the water seems inviting.
Some part of our being knows this is where we came from. We
long to return, and we can, because the cosmos is also within us.
We're made of star stuff. We are a way for the cosmos to know
itself.

When you are finished with the loving kindness blessings, spend
a few moments thinking about what you have just done before
carrying on with your meditation or the rest of your day or evening.
You may even wish to write about your experience in your journal.

These loving kindness blessings are recited by members of the
Marin Sangha, led by Philip Moffitt. I enjoyed them so much I
wanted to share them with you.

Alternative Loving Kindness Blessings

You can use the verses in the previous section, or you can make up
your own. Here is another set of verses you may want to use from
time to time.

May you be at peace.
May your heart remain open.
May you know the beauty and the radiance of your own true
nature.
May you be healthy.
May you be free and happy, truly happy.

This was the second set of verses for loving kindness blessings
that I learned back in 1990. The traditional set of verses goes like
this:

May you be happy.
May you be well.
May you be safe.
May you be peaceful and at ease.

The first set of verses that I learned were the traditional ones the rabbis would say at the end of services on the Sabbath and Jewish holidays:

May the Lord bless you and keep you;
May the Lord's face shine upon you and be gracious to you;
May the Lord's face lift towards you and place upon you peace.

While we are on the subject of loving kindness meditation I want to share with you a beautiful song a friend of my shared with me for healing, relaxation, and inner peace. The song is sung by Ashana in an album called *All is Forgiven*. It goes like this:

Loving kindness
For All Beings
From the ONE beyond the stars
Through the darkness
Into the light
We behold the gift of peace

This song moves me every time I listen to it. I used it exclusively when I was undergoing my recent cancer treatments.

For more information about this type of meditation, please visit **Meditation Practices**[4] and search for *"loving kindness."*

GRATITUDE MEDITATION

Research has shown that the practice of gratitude can increase your happiness by a considerable amount – as much as 25 percent! They say that you can develop a stronger immune system and lower your blood pressure. You will feel more states of positive emotions, have more joy, optimism, and happiness, and feel more generous and compassionate. Practicing gratitude will also reduce your feelings of loneliness and isolation.

The practice of gratitude in daily life takes the form of thanking people for what they do for you. It also involves taking the time to be kind and courteous to other people. This helps to spread gratitude to more people, and it sets up a "pay it forward" situation. It will help you strengthen your social ties that will increase your feeling of being interconnected.

Gratitude is also a very potent antidote to depression. This is because we realize that the world is not devoid of goodness, love, and kindness. Gratitude takes us out of ourselves.

There are many ways to express gratitude in addition to the meditation practice outlined below. One idea is to keep a gratitude journal. Make it a habit to write down or share with a loved one your thoughts about the gifts you've received each day.

Another idea is to write a thank-you note. You can make yourself happier and nurture your relationship with another person by writing a thank-you letter expressing your enjoyment and appreciation of that person's impact on your life. Send it, or better yet, deliver and read it in person if possible. Make a habit of sending at least one gratitude letter a month. Once in a while, write one to yourself.

If you find that you don't have time to write or visit your friend, it may help to think about that person and mentally thank them for being nice to you.

Zen Master Thich Nhat Hanh is always teaching us that happiness can only be found in the present moment and that we have everything we need to be happy here and now. He says that we can feel the warmth of the sun, the beauty of the flowers, the fragrance of the trees, the power of the mountains, and the peaceful calm of the mountain lake, reflecting the light of the moon. He calls these "the wonders of life." We can all be grateful for these wonders of life and find many more that appeal to us.

When my girls were young, they both had an insatiable desire for Barbie dolls, toys, clothing, and other worldly objects. When their craving was so strong that they made themselves (and us) unhappy, my wife would say to them, "To desire what you don't have is to waste what you do have."

This seemed to calm them down on occasions and it is forever implanted in their minds. Just recently, one of my daughters, now

32, realized just how blessed her childhood had been and she texted us a beautiful message about how grateful she was for having parents like us. You can believe that this thank-you note was one of the items for my gratitude meditation that night and the next morning.

There was a story from the time of the Buddha that moved me tremendously. I am indebted to H.E. Tulku Yeshi Rinpoche for this story.

A poor man asked the Buddha,
"Why am I so poor?"
The Buddha said, "You did not learn to give."
So the poor man said, "But, if I don't have anything to give?"
The Buddha said, "You have a few things:
The Face, which can give a smile;
The Mouth, you can praise or comfort others;
The Heart, it can open up to others;
The Eyes, they can look at the other with the eyes of compassion;
The Body, which can be used to help others."

You can find a recording of this on **Meditation Practices**[4].

Gratitude Meditation Practice

The gratitude meditation practice can be combined with the loving kindness meditation practice or precede or follow the mindfulness of breathing meditation practice. It can also be done quite alone and often during the day as things are happening in your life.

I do this practice before I go to sleep, and when I awake. Also, many times during the day, I take note of something that I am grateful for.

The stand-alone practice begins with taking a comfortable position on a chair or cushion or lying down. If you are lying down, try not to fall asleep!

Step 1: Begin the practice by taking a minimum of three deep breaths. As you breathe in, follow your in breath all the way in. As you breathe out, follow your out breath all the way out.

Step 2: When you are ready, allow your breathing to become normal and withdraw yourself into yourself. Become aware of your meditation seat. Be aware of no other spaces but these spaces. Be aware of no other times but these times. Be here. Be now. Be here now.

Step 3: Bring to mind an event, object, or experience that happened today that you are truly grateful for. If you can't think of one, look back in your life and find something that you are truly grateful for.

It may be something as simple as a smile you received from someone while you were walking to or from work or the friendliness of a clerk that checked out your groceries, like in the story of the poor man. If you take notice of these kinds of acts of kindness, you will soon find yourself "paying it forward."

Now acknowledge your gratitude and feel the joy you had when the event, object, or experience took place.

Step 4: Repeat the above at least two more or as many times as you want.

Do this every day for maximum benefit.

For more information about this type of meditation, please visit **Meditation Practices**[4] and search for "*gratitude.*"

FORGIVENESS MEDITATION

Forgiveness is the complementary practice to gratitude. This is because it is often more difficult to forgive some than to be grateful for something someone else has done. Also, if you have not forgiven yourself or another person, you will find it difficult to shower them with loving kindness blessings.

Often, the difficulty arises because you have not forgiven yourself for your past thoughts, words, and actions and you are holding onto them, perhaps because you feel undeserving.

But take this to heart. The act of forgiving yourself can free you from a lot of suffering. The past is already gone and you can do nothing about it. The future has not yet come so you cannot do anything about it either. We only have the present moment in which to experience the wonders of life.

So part of the forgiveness practice is to first of all, forgive ourselves. I know this may sound hard to do, but with diligence and effort, it is totally possible.

They say that time heals all wounds, but the only time we have is right now. Therefore, forgiveness and the happiness that comes from it are all available in the present moment.

In the words of Jack Kornfield, an eminent meditation teacher, author, and co-founder of the Spirit Rock Meditation Center, "Forgiveness is giving up all hope of a better past!"

Sometimes, it is very difficult to forgive, especially ourselves or someone close to us. We often forget that the act that someone else did to us that we have not yet forgiven was done from a place of fear or anger or both. The oThe action could have come from the other person as a cry for help. The act may have been done from an experience of suffering.

Perhaps it makes sense to forgive the person and not forgive the act. For example, if someone knows that their partner has been unfaithful, they can learn to forgive their partner, but not their infidelity.

Sometimes, a prayer of forgiveness comes spontaneously into your heart as it did in mine on August 5, 2012 in Central Park, New York City. I was walking with my son, his mother Linda, and his girlfriend (now his fiancé), Ashley when we got the idea to honor the death of my mother by going to a Jewish deli for dinner. The previous night, we remembered Linda's father in a different Jewish deli.

I called my sister to get the exact date of my mother's passing in August of 1987. When she shocked me with the news that my brother was in the hospital in Santa Monica, California, I had to sit down to absorb her statement. Without any further thought, I prayed for my brother's rapid recovery and dropped all the resentment I had been carrying for umteen years. I spontaneously forgave him for everything. We are talking again as he continues to recover from a serious illness, and he even came to visit me in April, 2014.

From then on, he became one of the people that I showered loving kindness blessings on in Step 6 of the loving kindness meditation practice. I keep in touch with his healing process with frequent telephone calls.

Forgiveness Meditation Practice

The forgiveness meditation practice has three components. The first component is to ask for forgiveness from people we may have harmed. The second component is to forgive ourselves. The third component is to forgive others.

It is important to note that if we are not comfortable with any of the components or all of them, we do not have to force ourselves to do the practice. For example, if we feel we cannot forgive ourselves, we can sit quietly and look deeply to see if there is a tiny element of forgiveness that we can muster for something we did in our lives. We can look for a tiny spark that can open our hearts for forgiveness.

Similarly, if we find that we cannot forgive a certain other person, because what they "did to us" was so unforgivable, we can sit quietly and look for a tiny opening in our heart to that person. Maybe we can find a small morsel of forgiveness and forgive them for part of their actions.

Maybe, with practice, these tiny sparks and these tiny openings can blossom into a full-fledged heart opening and we can truly begin to forgive. Perhaps, there is a small offense that you no longer wish to hold onto and can use that as a lever to pry open your heart.

These small little openings can lead to full-on forgiveness if we are diligent and practice with enough patience to allow them to flower.

This practice again begins with taking a comfortable position on a chair or cushion or lying down. If you are lying down, try not to fall asleep! If you are uncomfortable with one of the components of forgiveness, skip it until you are ready to deal with it. For example, if there is someone you cannot possibly forgive right now, use another person or situation. If you can't think of anyone to forgive, begin by forgiving yourself.

Step 1: Begin the practice by taking a minimum of three deep breaths. As you breathe in, follow your in breath all the way in. As you breathe out, follow your out breath all the way out.

Step 2: When you are ready, allow your breathing to become normal and withdraw yourself into yourself. Become aware of your meditation seat. Be aware of no other spaces but these spaces. Be aware of no other times but these times. Be here. Be now. Be here now.

Step 3: As your breathing becomes normal, begin to feel what it feels like to have your heart closed to forgiving yourself or others. Now, as you are sitting or lying there feeling all of this emotion, recall a time when you felt that you had harmed someone in ways that were hurtful and not necessarily intentional.

As you recall this time allow yourself to visualize the way you hurt that person. Feel the pain that you inflicted due to your own confusion and suffering.

Now simply ask for forgiveness by saying to that person, "Please forgive me. Please release me. I'm sorry that I caused you pain."

Alternatively, you can use these more elaborate phrases for asking for forgiveness from others:

> There are many ways I have harmed you, knowingly and unknowingly – betrayed you, abandoned you, caused you pain so many times. I remember these now and feel the sorrows I still carry.

> In the many ways I have hurt or harmed you, betrayed you, caused you suffering, out of my own fear and confusion, out of my own pain, anger and hurt and misunderstanding, in this moment, I ask your forgiveness. I ask your forgiveness. Please forgive me. Please forgive me. May I be forgiven.[15]

If the situation that you are recalling is too difficult for you to confront at this time, be sure to forgive yourself for not being able to let it go right now. You can also choose someone that is much easier to forgive and then build up to forgiving the difficult person.

Step 4: Take another deep breath or two to give yourself the time to release whatever charge is left over from Step 3. Then recall a time when you have hurt yourself or did something to yourself that you feel sorry for.

When you have recalled such a time, think to yourself, "I have caused myself pain and suffering for this and other thoughts, words, or actions. I now forgive myself." You may wish to repeat this several times, either by recalling other events or staying with the time that you recalled.

If this step seems too difficult, tune into your feelings and try to discover what is going on. Forgive yourself for a small thing to get started, and progress gently and compassionately to what you once thought to be unforgivable.

Step 5: Again, take one or more deep breaths to relieve yourself of the feelings and sensation that arose when you were forgiving yourself. Then, recall a time when another person caused you to suffer, either by words or actions.

Try to make this recollection as vivid as possible and bring to mind the feelings you have about it. Then remember that the person who you recalled was also suffering knowingly or unknowingly when she or he caused you harm.

Now pick a small part of this pain and say to the person, "I forgive you. I release you." Repeat this as many times as needed.

Each time you return to this forgiveness meditation, allow forgiveness to arise little by little until you feel free.

For more information about this type of meditation, please visit **Meditation Practices**[4] and search for *"forgiveness."*

MINDFUL EATING

Most of us rush through our meals without thinking about our food or even tasting it! It goes in. We feel full. We leave the table. Done!

This is not the right way to eat. This is no way to enjoy our meals. What we need to do is to eat mindfully.

What is mindful eating? Mindful eating is the practice of paying attention to each bite of food you take. It is contemplating the origin of the food. We think about such questions as, where did it come from? How did it get here? Who raised the food for us? What were the circumstances under which it was raised?

These days, we even might want to consider whether the food has gluten in it or not. We also want to avoid genetically modified organisms (GMO) and only buy non-GMO food.

We might want to reduce or eliminate animal and animal products from our diet to reduce the suffering of living beings and preserve our planet. Did you know that the major cause of global warming is due to greenhouse gases from animal waste products, especially methane? This amounts to 51% of global warming when you consider all the destruction of the rainforests, soil degradation, and animal waste products. Did you know that the amount of water you use for one year of daily showers is the amount of water needed to raise just one pound of beef?

We might want to express gratitude to the producers of the food and recognize and transform our unwholesome thoughts, especially greed (putting more than we can eat on our plate). We might want to learn to eat in moderation.

When I saw Michael Broffman at the beginning of the 2013 episode of muscle invasive bladder cancer, he told me about three categories of eating food.

The first category he called the science of eating. This involves scientifically being mindful of nutrition, carbs, gluten, and whether or not the food contains GMO's or is organic.

The second category has to do with the preparation of food. This is the artistic approach. The considerations here are the attitudes of the people preparing the food and how they are putting their energy into it.

The third category is the context of eating. What this means is that if you are enjoying a meal prepared by a friend or a nice restaurant, it hardly matters what you eat. Unless, of course, you are on a gluten-free diet or have other important restrictions.

Keep these categories in mind as you learn more about mindfulness in eating.

Mindful Eating Practices

When we slow down and eat mindfully, our life and health takes on a much deeper quality. Being present with every bite benefits us physically, emotionally, and spiritually. We feel nourished on all levels and this has a significant influence on the rest of our day.

If you want to improve your life and health, physically, and mentally, try these five practices for mindful eating. You may want to adopt one of them per week to see how they work for you and then choose the ones that you relate to best.

1. **Slow down** and enjoy every minute of your meal. Eat slowly by chewing every bite at least 30 times before swallowing.
2. **Plan a healthy diet** around non-GMO organic fruits and vegetables. If you must eat meat, make sure it is organic, free range, and that the animals have not been fed GMO foods. I enjoy fresh fish from the farmer's market, often.
3. **Completely avoid** soft drinks of any kind, alcoholic

beverages, and GMO foods. Soft drinks contain too much sugar. Diet soft drinks are even worse, for they often contain the poison, aspartame. It has been shown that artificial sweetening signals the brain that real sugar is coming, which it never does. This puts your whole system on red alert, waiting for the promised real energy boost. As for GMO foods, no one really knows the long-term effects of these foods on your body.

4. **Between each bite**, put down your fork, spoon, or sandwich while you chew each bite of food completely.

5. **Be grateful** for the food that is on your table. Contemplate the interconnections that had to be made for you to have food on your table.

You might enjoy the following contemplations before eating. They come from Zen Master Thich Nhat Hanh and the monks and nuns of Plum Village. They are recited at meals and retreats.

This food is the gift of the whole universe: the earth, the sky, numerous living beings, and much hard, loving work.
May we eat with mindfulness and gratitude so as to be worthy to receive it.
May we recognize and transform our unwholesome mental formations, especially our greed, and learn to eat with moderation.
May we keep our compassion alive by eating in such a way that we reduce the suffering of living beings, preserve our planet, and reverse the process of global warming.
We accept this food so that we may nurture our sisterhood and brotherhood, strengthen our community and nourish our ideal of serving all living beings.

Mindful eating is also a way to promote weight loss. When you eat mindfully, you may learn not to eat more than you absolutely need, and you may be able to recognize that you are full sooner.

At one of our meetings of the **Mindfulness in Healing**[1] sangha (meditation group) in 2014, one lovely participant brought in a basket of freshly picked oranges with their stems in place. She wrapped the stems with a red ribbon.

After our invocation and thirty minutes of mindful meditation, we practiced not-eating meditation with the oranges. They were not yet ripe for eating.

We picked up our oranges and felt the texture of their skins. We noticed the flower-like structure at the junction of the stem and the skin. We noticed places on the stem where possibly other orange flowers could have developed.

On the orange, itself, we noticed the rough skin and indentations here and there. We scratched the surface of the orange skin in order to smell its fragrant citrus odor. We placed the orange next to our ear to hear the wind blowing in the tree where the orange grew.

We did a guided meditation of what it would fell like to peel the orange, all in one piece. We could experience what the rind felt like. We could feel the moisture of the orange juice inside. We could experience the thrill of breaking out one segment and tasting its sweet flavor.

Everyone was delighted by this experience. You can try these steps the next time you eat an orange or tangerine. You will also be delighted.

SOUND MEDITATION PRACTICES

Before we move on to contemplative meditation practices, it is important to note that there are dozens of different meditation practices that you can learn and enjoy. The bottom line is it is much more important to meditate daily than it is to be fixed on a single meditation practice.

Mantra Meditation

One of the more common meditation practices that is used today involves a sound or a word or a phrase - a **mantra** - that is repeated over and over again to enhance your concentration. Referring to the poem at the beginning of Chapter 1, my mantra since then has been "Healthy... Free." When I breathe in, I think "Healthy." When I breathe out, I think, "Free" – free of cancer.

When I place my left foot while waking, I think, "Healthy." When I place my right foot while walking, I think, "Free."

These practices have nurtured my well-being for more than

eighteen years.

I am pleased to say that one of the most powerful meditation sessions I ever had in my life was doing mantra meditation. This occurred in 1973 when I was studying in the Ozark Mountains in Arkansas with Father Eli. It was early in my training there and I was still practicing yoga and mantra meditation.

I had received the mantra the year before when I was studying at the feet of Swami Rama of the Himalayas and Dr. Arya (now, Swami Veda Bharati, who also passed away recently) outside of Chicago, Illinois. I had so many mind-blowing experiences with these two teachers you'll probably wonder why I didn't continue with them.

I was living at that time in Evanston, Illinois with my first wife and son and teaching at the local community college. One evening I went to an occult book store expecting a talk on yoga and meditation. I must have gotten the night wrong for there was Father Eli telling wisdom stories that captivated my attention. I tried to get up and leave, but somehow I just couldn't.

I returned monthly for several months and began to feel an affinity for the wisdom teachings he was talking about. They all made sense to me and I was eager to learn more.

When two of his students who were travelling with him with their young child needed a place to stay, I offered my home. My wife and son were off to California with her new boyfriend.

One of them initiated me into the meditation practices that are taught by Father Eli. I felt a strange sense of familiarity with it because it was so similar to what I learned in the Silva Mind Control course which I took two or three years earlier. You can read more about the Silva Life System on **Meditation Practices**[4].

The next month, Father Eli invited me to train with him in the summer. I spent three weeks deliberating this decision while I was negotiating a clean financial break with my first wife.

So there I was, sitting in my van on the land owned by Father Eli in the Ozark Mountains, practicing my mantra. I entered into a divine state of meditation where I experienced that I was empty of a separate self. Then, a feeling of bliss that ensued for what seemed like a long time filled my mind and body. I was refreshed and excited to learn all I could from Father Eli.

This experience was proof to me that meditation furthers one's development on the path to well-being.

When you do mantra meditation, you can choose one of the classical mantras like, "Om," or "Om Mane Padme Hum" (Oh! The jewel in the lotus). Or choose something of your own liking. I like, for example, the words of Ashana's song, "Loving kindness for all beings."

The second most common type of sound meditation is called *kirtan*, or devotional chanting. This type is familiar to all of us who have ever heard the beautiful voice of Krishna Das or Jai Uttal. It is entirely similar to Gregorian chants and other Christian modes of devotional singing.

Binaural Beats

The sound meditation you are going to learn about now is moving very fast on the popularity charts, but hasn't reached the mainstream. This type is called *binaural beats* or binaural tones. Binaural beats can induce a state of deep relaxation and meditation if composed properly.

Binaural beats occur when two sound frequencies are directed separately to each ear. For example, if a note of 440 HZ (this is actually A above middle C) is sent to the left ear and 450 HZ is sent to the right ear. The 10 HZ frequency difference is heard by the brain as a binaural beat.

These binaural beat frequencies correspond to different brain wave frequency ranges. Binaural beat frequencies of

- Less than 4 HZ: delta waves and correspond to states of dreamless sleep with loss of body awareness
- 4-7 HZ: theta waves and correspond to deep relaxation and meditative states as well as non-REM (random eye movement) sleep
- 8-12 HZ: mu waves and correspond to sensorimotor rhythm
- 7-13 HZ: alpha waves and correspond to relaxation while awake, states of drowsiness before and after sleep, REM sleep and the dream state.
- 13-39 HZ: beta waves and correspond to the normal levels of experience
- Greater than 40 HZ: gamma waves and correspond to

higher mental activity, including problem solving, perception, and consciousness

If you want to experiment with binaural beats, you can visit YouTube and search for "binaural beats."

CONTEMPLATIONS

We conclude this chapter with a selection of contemplations that you can incorporate into your daily mindfulness practice as you see fit. All of the contemplative meditations begin with finding a comfortable position on your cushion, straight-back chair or lying down and taking a minimum of three deep breaths. Then withdraw yourself into yourself and begin the contemplation exercise.

The Five Remembrances

The five remembrances are practiced daily by monks and nuns, lay men and lay women all over the world. You don't have to be a Buddhist to practice them. They have universal application for all beings.

The first time you read them, you may have a little difficulty, but as you get used to them, you will realize their inherent truth. Their truth is self-evident and you will gain a lot of insight by practicing them.

The five remembrances are:

I am of the nature to grow old – I cannot escape old age.
I am of the nature to have ill health – I cannot escape ill health.
I am of the nature to die – I cannot escape death.
Everyone I love and everything I have are of the nature to change –
I cannot escape the impermanence of all things.
My actions are my only true belongings - I cannot escape the
consequences of my actions. My actions are the ground upon
which I stand.

The way to practice the five remembrances is as follows. Read the first verse carefully and make sure you understand the content. It is obvious that everyone and everything grows old.

As you breathe in, think to yourself, "I am of the nature to grow old." As you breathe out, think to yourself, "I cannot escape old age." After repeating this to yourself several time, and when you are sure of the truth of its teaching, you can simplify the practice a little.

As you breathe in, think to yourself, "Old age," or "Growing old." As you breathe out, think to yourself, "No escape." Follow this short cut only if it appeals to you and if you want to do it.

In either format, repeat the phrase or short cut a minimum of ten times or for five minutes, or whatever feels comfortable to you.

Then repeat this process for each of the other remembrances.

The short-cut versions are

Old age – No escape.
Ill health –No escape.
Death – No escape.
Impermanence – No escape.
Actions – No escape.

Impermanence

After practicing these for a while, you may begin to have a deep insight into the reality of impermanence. This is one of the fundamental laws of nature and it is also true in the natural world. We would not be here if things were not impermanent.

We are here because of the explosions of several supernovae in our region of the galaxy. Supernovae are large stars that create the heave elements necessary for life as they grow old, burn all of their nuclear fuel, and die in a massive explosion. Supernovae explosions in galaxies far away are so bright that they outshine their whole galaxies.

Out of the mass of supernovae debris in this part of the galaxy, our sun was born and the planets and moons with it about 4.6 billion years ago. The earth developed to what it is today by absorbing the impact of planetesimals (small planet-like objects) and other objects of various sizes.

Life developed on earth about 3.6 billion years ago, and humans made their first appearance as recently as 2.5 million years ago. On this cosmic scale of things, human life is just a baby!

Scientists predict that even the sun will die – in about 5-6 billion years. The sun will become a "red giant" star, become much hotter, and expand greatly. It will engulf Mercury, Venus, and yes, even the whole Earth. The only remnant of human life will be somewhere in outer space where the Voyager 1 and Voyager 2 are still roaming around in the vast emptiness of space.

So you see, instead of wanting things to be permanent, we should celebrate impermanence and shout, "Long live impermanence!"

To contemplate impermanence, begin with several deep breaths as before. Withdraw yourself into yourself and become aware of your meditation seat. Bring your attention to your breathing.

When you are settled down in your breathing, begin to notice sensations in your body. You can do this by scanning your body from head to toes or from toes to head. Or you can do this by just noting sensations anywhere in your body.

Notice how sensations come into being, stay for a while, and leave. For example, you may have an itch on your arm. Your first impulse is to scratch the itch for immediate relief. However, if you allow it to just be for a moment or two, you will notice that it will change and most likely dissipate.

All of these changing sensations anywhere in your body are impermanent. There is nothing to get hung up about.

No Permanent Self

What more can we learn from the insight of impermanence? Well, if everything is changing, then there is nothing for us to call our permanent self. Furthermore, within our bodies and within our minds, there is nothing that lasts for more than a moment. Therefore nothing could be identified as the unchanging self or soul.

Nonetheless, it still makes sense to talk about ourselves as if we have some semblance of permanence. That's why we say such things as, "I am of the nature to grow old." This "I" is a conventional way of referring to our specific incarnation in this universe at this moment.

To contemplate no permanent self, begin with several deep breaths as before. Withdraw yourself into yourself and become aware of your meditation seat. Bring your attention to your breathing.

When you are settled down in your breathing, ask yourself the following questions.

"Are my eyes or what I see myself?"

"Are my ears or what I hear myself?

"Is my nose or the odors I smell myself?"

"Is my tongue or what I taste myself?"

"Is my skin or tactile sensations myself?"

"Is my mind or brain myself?"

"Are my thoughts, memories, plans, images, hopes and dreams myself?"

"If none of these sense doors or sensations is me, what am I?"

Ponder these questions as long as you want. Then take several deep breaths to return to your daily life or drift off to sleep.

Interbeing

Once we grasp the ideas of impermanence and no permanent self (non-self), we begin to realize that nothing we know of has a separate existence. You cannot be by yourself, alone. I cannot be by myself, alone. We all have to inter-be with each other and the whole cosmos. The insight of Interbeing means that we are interconnected with everything around us, near and far. We all have to recognize that our existence depends upon the existence of others and the whole earth around us.

We depend on others to bring food to our tables. We depend on others to build housing for us. We depend on others to make clothing so that we won't freeze to death in the winter. Our dependence on everything around us is so deeply engrained that we hardly even notice it.

Have you thought about how that piece of corn you are eating arrived on your plate? Who planted the seed? Who harvested it? Who brought it to the market? Who purchased it? Who provided the energy for you to cook the corn? When you think about it, it takes a lot of people and causes and conditions to bring a single ear of corn to your dinner table.

Unsatisfactoriness

We all know that life is full of disappointments, complications, and unsatisfactoriness. When desirable things happen, we want them to last forever. When undesirable things happen, we want them to go away instantly. How do we reconcile these opposing forces?

When we try to hold onto something that is changing beyond

our control, we are bound to be disappointed and feel depressed. We identify suffering with unpleasant situations most of the time. However, pleasant ones can also lead to suffering when we become attached to them. The more we crave pleasant sensations, the more unhappiness they will bring. It is in the craving and grasping for pleasant sensations that suffering abides.

Both pleasant experiences and unpleasant experiences are of the nature to change. They are impermanent, ever changing, and cause us misery. Coming to terms with this can bring on equanimity.

A funny thing happened a moment ago which illustrates this point. None of my friends with whom I attend the Dean Lectures on astronomy at the California Academy of Sciences were available to go with me tonight. So I thought I would get clever. I made a call to a couple that I am acquainted with who normally attend the lectures. The number I had for them had been disconnected.

I knew that the wife of the couple plays tennis at a local tennis club and decided to call there. I had played there many times in tennis competitions. It just so happened that the person I wanted to talk to was at the club at this time. I was elated.

After getting her phone numbers into my contacts, I asked if she and her husband were going to the lecture tonight. She said that they had grandparent duty and would not be going. I was deflated.

A few minutes later, I checked the internet to see what the topic of the talk would be and decided that it was not so interesting that I wanted to go alone.

So, within the space of a few minutes, I had a pleasant experience (i.e., finding my friend at the tennis club), and unpleasant experience (i.e., she and her husband not going), and a neutral experience (i.e., deciding not to go). The whole thing vanished and I continued working on my writing.

The contemplation of unsatisfactoriness is begun the way the others are – with at least three deep breaths. This is followed by bringing your attention into the body. When you are ready, begin the following contemplation.

Recall a time when you were disappointed with something that happened in your life. Make it a small disappointment at first so you can get used to doing the contemplation.

Recall how you felt about the situations. What did it feel like?

Did it make you feel more than disappointed, like miserable? Did you get depressed? Notice your feelings.

Now pay attention primarily to how the situation made you want to avoid experiences like this. Notice the flavor of the avoidance. Do you see how we want to avoid unpleasant experiences?

How long did it last? Were you able to recognize that this unpleasant experience was impermanent?

Take a full deep breath or two as you let this experience go and be just what it is. How do you feel now? What sensations are you experiencing right now?

Now recall a time when you were elated with something that happened. Again, make it a small event that you can practice with until you become familiar with the contemplation.

Recall how you felt in this situation. What did it feel like? Did you want the make the experience last and last? Notice whether you wanted it to last.

Recall how long this experience lasted. Wasn't it also impermanent? Didn't you want more?

The wanting more of this experience is craving. Craving is an aspect of pleasant experiences when we want more.

How did you feel about the experience of elation? Did it give you more energy? Were you happy about it?

When you are ready, take a deep breath or two and let this experience go and be just what it is.

Now you have an opportunity to compare the unsatisfactory experience with the satisfactory experience. How do they compare? Are you able to let both experiences be just as they are without craving the good one and being adverse to the bad one? When this happens, you naturally experience a state of equanimity.

When you are ready, return to your normal life. You now have the experience of knowing that both pleasant and unpleasant experiences are impermanent and they pass.

7 REACH OUT TO OTHERS

Gathering your friends and family around you for support is one of the most valuable actions you can take to begin your recovery. This can be very healing.

Your people can help you with meals, transportation, and support. They will be happy to pick up your prescriptions or help you with your children. They will come to your house and sit with you or visit you at the clinic while you are having chemotherapy.

I found that inviting people over for a potluck followed by a period of silent sitting meditation was powerful.

I remember two significant events during 1997 that touched me deeply. The first was in early March. I really didn't think I would make it, but somehow I got to attend my son's performance as Marcello in *La Boheme* in Santa Cruz, California.

Since Micah was eleven, he has been interested in music and acting. At that time, he joined the San Francisco Boys Chorus, which he participated in for more than ten years. In high school, he was a founding member of the Barber Shop Quartet and had leading roles in many plays like *The Fantastics* (his senior project) and *West Side* Story. At Stanford University, he was the leader of an a Capella group, *The Fleet Street Singers*, and took part in many productions.

After a busy day with the doctors, we drove down to Capitola and I took a nap before the performance. During dinner, Micah seemed really calm for a person playing a leading role in a major opera. Watching his performance, I felt a lot of joy and was able to keep thoughts of cancer out of my mind.

The second event took place in June. My daughter, Rachael, graduated from eighth grade with a moving-on ceremony at a local church. On that day, she delivered what everyone thought was the most moving speech of the day. She praised Marin Horizon School for "how each student is considered an individual," with individual needs and different learning styles.

She had this to say about me:

"Last, but not least, my father, you have always been there for me even if you were going through rough times. You are so loving. You are the best father. I love you so much!"

After hearing this, my heart flew open and I felt the divine presence and wept for joy! She looked so beautiful in her fancy dress and I was so proud of the job she did.

Rachael got a degree in architecture and is now a yoga teacher, an Ayurveda practitioner and working for the Hoffman Institute.

With children like these, to give you much joy and happiness, it is no wonder I was able to heal from cancer.

Another event worth mentioning is the healing circle that took place just at the beginning of the 2013 episode. Seven friends, my wife, and Rachael gathered for a healing circle led by two of my most powerful friends.

Ramona is a Kundalini Yoga teacher and a good friend since 1988. She led the ceremony with Clare, a shaman specializing in rituals. They placed me lying down in the center of the circle with everyone else sitting around.

Clare began the circle by having each person say a few healing words to me. This brought tears to my eyes, a smile on my face, and laughter to the circle. The words people chose were very nourishing and touched me deeply.

Next, Ramona led us in a couple of Kundalini Yoga chants. This was followed by Clare working her magic.

I felt loved and accepted by everyone. They all had the best wishes for me and many stayed for a vegetarian curry dish for dinner. I am totally grateful to everyone who came and to those who were invited but could not come.

SUPPORT GROUPS

Another thing to consider, which may be just as important as spending time with your family and friends, is to investigate support groups in your area. Dr. Daniel Goleman has reported that participating in support groups extends longevity by as much as 50%.

At support groups, you'll find people with your same or similar condition and you can learn a lot from their stories. They can share with the group what is going on in their treatment and this may help you to gain insight into what you may have in store for you.

In some situations, this can be frightening, but I think it is better to know than to be surprised later. Many times, you'll learn the answers to questions you forgot to ask your doctor or didn't know to ask your doctor.

For example, I learned in a support group early during my first episode with bladder cancer that chemotherapy sometimes produces a kind of neuropathy in some parts of your body. I was forewarned and forearmed and I was lucky enough not to have any.

I found support groups so important in my healing experience that I started one of my own! This was part of my effort to give back to my community (see *Give Back – Chapter 9*) and to make what I had learned available to others. This book is also part of that effort.

The Center for Attitudinal Healing

During my recovery, I attended several different support groups. One of them was at the Center for Attitudinal Healing founded by Dr. Gerald Jampolsky, MD. While I attended the life-threatened group, my wife attended the caregiver's group. Both of us learned a considerable amount from our respective groups. On the ride home we would share insights and good news as well as stories of tragedy.

The Center for Attitudinal Healing is based on Dr. Jampolsky's book, *Love is Letting Go of Fear*[16] and the Principles of Attitudinal Healing:

1. *The essence of our being is love.*
2. *Health is inner peace. Healing is letting go of fear.*
3. *Giving and receiving are the same.*
4. *We can let go of the past and the future.*
5. *Now is the only time there is and each instant is for giving.*
6. *We can learn to love ourselves and others by forgiving rather than judging.*
7. *We can become love finders rather than fault finders.*
8. *We can choose and direct ourselves to be peaceful inside regardless of what is happening outside.*
9. *We are students and teachers to each other.*
10. *We can focus on the whole of life rather than the fragments.*
11. *Since love is eternal death need not be viewed as fearful.*
12. *We can always perceive ourselves and others as either extending love or giving a call for help.*

Anna Halprin

One of the most important and influential groups I attended was Anna Halprin's cancer support group which was held at Marin General Hospital in Greenbrae, California and in Anna's studio in Kentfield, California.

Anna Halprin is a cancer survivor, and is still teaching today at the age of 95. She was the winner of the Isadora Duncan Award in 1997 and many, many others before and after that. Each year around the beginning of June, she leads a world-wide dance event called, "Planetary Dance: A Call for Peace."

Each week, we would meet and Anna would have a theme for that week. She would play music and we would dance to the theme she had presented.

Next, we would draw something using cray-pas on a big sheet of paper. The drawing was supposed to express our feelings from the dance and about the theme. Some of these drawings are in my book, *Stop Cancer in its Tracks: Your Path to Mindfulness in Healing Yourself³*.

In 2007, Anna received the California Pacific Medical Center Pioneer Award in Integrative Medicine from the Institute for Health and Healing. I attended the event with my wife at the invitation from one of our friends.

I walked into the foyer on that cold wintery night (as cold as it gets in San Francisco) and there she was standing all by herself. I walked over to greet her, and suddenly she exclaimed, "Jerome – you're still alive!"

Needless to say, we had a wonderful time and I was invited to serve on the Community Council of the Institute for Health and Healing, who sponsored the event (see *Give Back* – Chapter 9).

Leslie Davenport's Group

Leslie Davenport offered a support group through California Cancer Care, where I had my chemotherapy and radiation.

We would meet in a small conference room with a table. It was usually a rather small group, say eight to twelve people.

We began with a guided imagery and proceeded to make a simple drawing about our experience. Then we would begin the process of checking in. We'd state our names and our conditions and then say whatever we felt like sharing. This part of Leslie's group was fairly typical of the other groups I attended.

It is my recommendation that you search out support groups relevant to your condition. Hearing other peoples' situations can inspire your own healing as well as help you come to terms with it.

Sometimes, what other people say may be frightening, but their experiences could lead you to asking specific questions of your medical team that you would not have thought of on your own. At other times, their positive results can set up a feedback mechanism in your psyche that stimulates your recovery process.

MEDITATION GROUPS

Meditation groups, such as **Mindfulness in Healing**[1] - the one I lead at the Pine Street Clinic in San Anselmo, can be of tremendous value, especially if you have decided to embark on a daily mindfulness practice. These groups allow you to connect with other people who are interested in meditation and everyone seems to benefit from group meditation.

A typical session in such groups consists of a period of sitting meditation which can be anywhere from fifteen to forty-five minutes, a lesson from the wisdom teachings, questions and answers, and an opportunity to share what is going on in your practice.

Mindfulness in Healing Sangha

Inspired by what I read in Daniel Goleman's book, *Emotional Intelligence*[17], I started meeting with people of all ages and all conditions in the lobby of the Pine Street Clinic in San Anselmo, California. I invited my dharma sister, Carolyn de Fay, LCSW to help me co-facilitate the group, and we have been meeting ever since. The group is called the **Mindfulness in Healing**[1] sangha and it was founded on the summer solstice of 2009. The people at Pine Street have been so generous with the use of their lobby space and we have been meeting there almost every week.

Please don't get stuck on the word, *sangha*. It is just a word that refers to a community of practitioners such as in a meditation group. When I can't be there, Carolyn leads. When Carolyn can't be there, I lead. When we are both there, we share the leadership role.

It is open to people with all types of healing needs on a drop in basis as well as their support persons. There is no charge, but donations to Pine Street are encouraged. Please feel free to join us if you are in the neighborhood.

Many people come just to meditate with us. In one case, the spouse of a person going through cancer came to us for over a year. Even though the other spouse passed away, the person who attended our group learned how to cope with the situation and continues to express gratitude for the help received.

Compassionate listening and loving speech are the foundations of our sharing practice. As mindfulness deepens awareness of our experience we find new ways to enhance our own well-being. We become able to transform our suffering and find freedom in the present moment, embracing a feeling of wellness.

We offer guided meditation and relaxation exercises to help promote a calm, clear mind and a peaceful, loving heart. This energy supports us in accepting our challenges just as they are and leads to an increased sense well-being and wellness.

We begin with an invocation:

This life is the gift of the whole Universe – the earth, the sky, and many generations.
May we live in mindfulness in order to enjoy the wonders of life."

Zen Master Thich Nhat Hanh teaches that the wonders of life can only be found in the present moment. Participating in a meditation group can help you to dwell happily in the present moment. The invocation is based on his writings and teachings, but the sitting group is nonsectarian.

The invocation is usually followed by a thirty-minute period of silent meditation. The members seem to really love this and find it to be beneficial to practice in a group setting.

We follow this with either sharing our practice, discussion on some meditation topic, or study of some text that will increase our understanding of our practice.

Shabbat Gathering

For more almost two years now, Mala and I have been attending a Shabbat gathering on the first Friday night of the month at the home of our good friends, Maryanne and David.

Our purpose of getting together is to build a loving community so that we can all thrive together. Each month, the love and trust we have for each other grows substantially. One of the nice things is that we share our friends in other contexts.

After several months of experimentation, we have come up with a format that we all love. We begin at 7:00 with a fifteen minute meditation. Sometimes one of us guides the group, but mostly we are on our own. Sitting silently in the presence of loving friends' supports our practice in many ways.

We come from different traditions or no tradition at all. It doesn't matter what you believe. Every tradition is welcome. Some of our members are practicing meditation for the first time.

After our meditation period, we have a potluck dinner. Even if you don't like to meditate, you would love to come for the dinner. It is always scrumptious and there is always plenty of food.

The third segment of our Shabbat gathering is a period of sharing. We pass a small blue ball around the room and people can share whatever they want. Everyone who is not talking is listening with deep presence and their full attention on the speaker. No one talks too long and this is because we tried timed three-minute periods for many months before dropping the timer.

Quite often, people share an experience of deep meaning to them and us. There is crying. There is laughter. There is presence. There is love and support.

On my birthday, I felt the love so strongly. They gave me a cup on a stand of angel wings. Each person had brought a little token of love and friendship for me to put in the cup. It sits on my desk and I am filled with love every time I look at it.

One Friday in April or May, we invited Anna Halprin to be with us. When it became her time to share, she told a story of great significance to me after my telling about the incident at the Institute for Health and Healing event in 2007.

She shared that she had stopped teaching cancer patients in 1997 because she had seen to many people pass away. This was too painful for her. When she saw me at the event, she was inspired once again to work with cancer patients. My survival had sparked her confidence in continuing her work with cancer patients.

Marin Sangha

The Marin Sangha was founded by meditation teacher Phillip Moffitt who is also the guiding teacher. He was once the CEO of Esquire Magazine and now he is a teacher of yoga and meditation.

Phillip is the author of two books, *Dancing With Life: Buddhist Insights for Finding Meaning and Joy in the Face of Suffering* and *Emotional Chaos to Clarity: How to Live More Skillfully, Make Better Decisions, and Find Purpose in Life*. He also is the founder and director of the Life Balance Institute where he trains organizational professionals on how to manage life transitions skillfully.

Marin Sangha is an insight meditation community that meets on Sunday nights from 6:00 to 8:00 PM at the St. Luke Presbyterian Church in San Rafael California. With over a hundred members, there is always someone to answer questions and guide new students.

Like the **Mindfulness in Healing**[1] sangha, the Marin Sangha operates on donations only. There is no charge for the teachings, but donations are accepted.

The schedule includes a forty-five minute silent meditation, which is sometimes guided, followed by ten to fifteen minutes of movement and a forty-five minute talk by various gifted teachers.

When I first started attending in 2009 or 2010, Phillip Moffitt was the primary teacher and was giving talks almost every week. Now, the teaching activities are shared by Phillip and others.

I stopped attending Marin Sangha in early 2012 because I came down with the flu and didn't want to infect anyone. Suddenly, I wasn't even thinking of going anymore, especially while I was managing cancer. Now, I look forward to going again and perhaps teaching there once or twice.

8 CREATE YOUR OWN MEDICAL TEAM

My team of medical doctors during the 1997 episode of bladder cancer included the urologist, Dr. Harry Neuwirth, MD; the oncologist, Dr. David Gullion, MD; the radiation oncologist, Dr. Francine Halberg, MD; and the family doctor, Dr. Robert Belknap, MD. This team worked together to give me the best possible standard medical treatment and I am very grateful to all of them. Even though the gold standard of medical care was to encourage me to have the radical cystectomy, their focus was on implementing the bladder sparing protocol and making sure that I was thriving.

When Dr. Neuwirth told me I had muscle invasive bladder cancer again in January 2014, he sent me immediately to see Dr. Maxwell Meng, MD, an outstanding surgeon at the University of California San Francisco (UCSF). He was the one in charge of my standard medical treatments. I also consulted Dr. Charles Ryan, MD, a medical oncologist at UCSF. These two doctors, along with Dr. Gullion and Dr. Neuwirth form my current team for standard medical treatment.

With the exception of Dr. Gullion, the rest of the team talked very little about alternative treatments. Dr. Gullion's practice included several of the methods discussed in the previous chapters including guided imagery, support groups, acupuncture, and Qi Gong. He is what I consider to be a medical expert and he would be suitable for many people dealing with cancer and needing chemotherapy.

What does it mean to create your own medical team and find a medical expert? It means to find a healing professional who knows about your situation and is knowledgeable about the standard medical treatments as well as possible alternatives for the illness you have.

Most people rely entirely on their doctors to know everything about their illness. They leave all the decisions to their doctors and follow blindly the standard medical treatments without question. They may ask questions of their doctors, but only to clarify their options, which may be limited.

In some cases, your primary doctor may be able to fulfill this role, providing he has an interest in recommending some of the alternatives discussed in previous chapters.

In our experiences, both present and past, we have found it beneficial to engage Michael Broffman, LAC. Don't be fooled by his lack of M. D. after his name. He is truly a multi-faceted genius who knows as much about standard medical treatments as he does about Chinese medicine, herbs, and acupuncture.

We first met Michael when our girls were in grade school in Mill Valley, California. His son was a year or two ahead of our oldest daughter.

When I was diagnosed with muscle invasive bladder cancer in 1997, we saw Michael within the first two weeks. He told us that bladder cancer is common in China and that there were alternatives to the standard medical treatment of radical cystectomy. He also said something that swayed my thinking away from radical cystectomy towards a bladder sparing protocol.

Michael told me that quite often people with replacement bladders often need additional surgery after about seven years. None of the doctors we consulted even came close to mentioning this little known fact! Dr. Peter Carroll, MD at UCSF and the rest of them all seemed to think that radical cystectomy was a "piece of cake," and there were very few side effects.

He also suggested that if the bladder sparing protocol failed, I could always resort to having the radical cystectomy at a later date. Here it is eighteen years later, and I still have my bladder!

A few days after this first meeting, Michael sent me a list of Chinese herbs and supplements that I should order and use during the chemotherapy and radiation that are part of the bladder sparing protocol. One of the most interesting things about this list was that each item was timed according to the stage of my treatment, which was divided three parts for each of two rounds of chemotherapy. The supplements I needed to take differed by round and part.

Part One was the first four days of chemotherapy. Michael wrote,

> *The essential effort during these several days is to enhance your circulation throughout your body. Chemotherapy drugs are dependent upon your blood circulation to carry it throughout your body. In this way it will encounter cancer cells wherever it goes. If*

there are areas of your body for whatever reason have poorer or less than optimal circulation than these areas will be somewhat undeserved by the chemotherapy. For example areas of your body where there has been previous surgery, scar tissues and injuries are areas where blood circulation may be inhibited. In addition areas of your body that you hold tension such as the lower back and neck may also be areas where circulation is poor. So the goal in part one is to use such techniques as imagery, visualizations and Qi-Gung to improve your circulation. Part One is a time to be restful, low key and minimize stress. Standing on line at the post office, being in traffic, entertaining and even watching the "news" may all be examples for you that counter your ability to relax.

Part two was the next seven days of chemotherapy. He wrote

At this time in your treatment the chemotherapy working very diligently on your behalf is killing numerous cells. These dead cells are piling up in your system and need to be removed. You do have organ systems that are well designed for this assignment; however the amount of dead cells accumulating often exceeds your natural ability to "cleanse" them out of your system. Therefore the main goal in this part is to assist your body in discharging and cleansing. In this way these dead cells will not be in the way of your next round of therapy. If you are doing imagery or visualizations then the emphasis shifts to address these new goals. As you will see in the herbal and supplement suggestions that follow, these shift also to adjust to this new part. Cleansing can also be figurative as well. Anything that you do during this part that helps you get rid of things is useful. For example, cleaning out closets and the garage, completing projects and unfinished and unresolved issues in your personal or business relationships.

Part three took into account the days between the chemotherapy rounds and after the chemotherapy was completed. Michael wrote,

During this time your blood counts will start to come up and much of your physiology will begin to normalize. You will feel better and start to have more energy than you felt in the previous

weeks. The goal at this time is to strengthen and enhance your immune system. Everything that you do should begin to reflect this. Engaging in activities that truly make you feel good and make you feel genuinely happy have a big priority at this time. If you can avoid using this time to "catch up" with activities and working overtime that is ideal.

With regard part one and "watching the news," I gave this up cold turkey. As you have seen when you read *Make Health-Promoting Lifestyle Changes*, watching the news usually violates the mindfulness training of mindful consumption.

Imagery, visualization, and tennis instead of Qi Gong were important activities during the whole treatment cycle, rather than only in part one. There were a few days where I didn't have the strength to play tennis, but on other occasions, I was quite fit.

In addition to timing the supplements and herbs according to the round and part of the chemotherapy, Michael recommended an ointment called *Mei-Po*, which is used in China to prevent and treat radiation burns. This cream worked extremely well for me, as did the supplements and herbs. The timing was so well coordinated with my treatment that I didn't lose my hair and didn't suffer radiation burns either.

Michael had many ideas for alternative treatments as well. For example, he thought that acupuncture would be beneficial during part three.

In addition to Michael Broffman's expertise, we also relied on the love and support from Dr. Martin Rossman, MD. Marty was the first physician to be licensed in acupuncture and he founded the Academy for Guided Imagery. Although he is not a cancer expert, he was one of the pioneers of integrative medicine and continues to be in practice today.

Marty visited me in the hospital on Super Bowl Sunday in 1997 and he provided me with a guided imagery tape that I used frequently during and after that first hospital stay. He attended the meeting we had with Dr. Neuwirth on the Friday after I left the hospital when he proclaimed my diagnosis of muscle invasive bladder cancer. (My research had shown me that this was one of the possibilities, and definitely not the best).

Throughout subsequent years, Marty has been a good friend and advisor. During the recent episode, Marty has treated me with acupuncture and guided imagery as well as served as my "primary doctor." We have also discussed in detail all of the alternative treatments that are under consideration.

If these wonderful practitioners are not enough, there are more medical experts in the field of alternative medicine that are now on my team. The first new person on my team is Dr. Sara Gordon, LAC, DAOM (doctor of oriental medicine.) She has become a beloved friend, like Marty and guided me to some supplements that I'm getting much benefit from.

The other person on my team is no stranger. We met Dr. Roger Morrison, MD, a medical doctor and leading homoeopathist, and when the girls were little, he treated them with homeopathy.

So, you see, we have been able to muster an excellent team of standard medical doctors and a team of excellent medical experts to take us through the trying time of cancer again.

This goes to show you how important it is to have medical experts involved as well as standard medical practitioners. Dr. Lissa Rankin, MD, states in her book *Mind over Medicine: Scientific Proof that You Can Heal Yourself*[8],

> *You may need more than just one person as you navigate the course of your treatment. You may need a whole team believing in you, offering you tools from their various toolboxes, and helping you make the body ripe for miracles. As you gather your team, you'll also need the members of that team to cooperate with one another.*

> *Acupuncturist Susan Fox calls such a team of collaborative practitioners "the healing round table." The healing round table is a collaborative process in which all health-care practitioners involved in the care of the patient are equal players whose opinions matter. At the healing round table, **the patient**, not the doctor, **presides** as the utmost authority. While physicians might be invited to the healing round table, the invitation to be present **does not grant doctors the right to give orders**, negate the advice of others at the table, or, most importantly, **disregard the***

patient's wishes.

This quote sums up my experience of creating my own medical team and facilitating the cooperation of all of the doctors and practitioners involved.

FINDING A MEDICAL EXPERT

I live in beautiful Marin County, California, just north of the Golden Gate Bridge. This area is known for its leadership in alternative medicine and many eminent practitioners also reside here.

Where you live may not be so well blessed with alternative medicine practitioners. Of course, you can call Michael Broffman or Dr. Marty Rossman for a consultation, but there is nothing like having someone in your own neighborhood that you can count on.

If you live in a large city, there are probably many practitioners in various fields of alternative medicine. Perhaps members of your family and friends can put you in touch with them.

As a last resort, you can look up practitioners by their professions. Here are some of the professions that could provide you with the alternative medical coaching and treatment that you need.

- Naturopaths
- Homeopaths
- Acupuncturists
- Masseuses
- Therapists
- Chiropractors
- Shamans
- Faith healers
- Ayurvedic practitioners

9 GIVE BACK

When you have recovered enough to spend time helping other people, you will find that you help yourself at the same time. Giving back to your community is a way to express gratitude for your healing experience.

If you have been excited by what you have read so far, then you know that many people have contributed to your sense of well-being and recovery. Your sense of well-being may have come from the standard medical treatments that you engaged in. But don't believe that it was the only source.

The alternative treatments you participated in (if any) had their effect on your recovery. So did the supplements you took and the lifestyle and diet changes you made. Perhaps your meditation practice helped you to be more calm about making decisions and confident in their results.

Now it is time to consider giving back you your community. You can volunteer to help out in the hospital where you were treated. You can let people know of your desire to give back to your community and they can recommend places where you may be able to serve. There are many things you can do.

Just six months after my first episode of muscle invasive bladder cancer in 1997, I offered a seminar at the hospital in which I had my surgery on Mindfulness and Art in Healing. In the class, we combined a guided meditation with movement and minor art projects.

In 2007, I was invited to serve on the Community Council of the Institute for Health and Healing (IHH) as a result of attending their fundraiser. That year, Anna Halprin was the winner of the Pioneer in Integrative Medicine award. That night, she delivered a stunning performance. You may recall from the *Reach Out to Others* chapter just how important Anna's contribution was to my healing.

At the same time I served at the IHH, I was also on the board of directors of the Marin AIDS Project. I held this position for the recommended three years and enjoyed everything about being there.

It was during this time in 2009 that I got the idea to branch out on my own. Having experienced the wonderful effects of several support groups, I came up with the idea of starting a group called,

Mindfulness in Healing (see *Reach Out to Others*).

During my most recent episode of cancer, I came across a wonderful woman who is giving back to her community. Her name is Karen Greene and she works at Sloan-Kettering in New York City. She is a survivor of metastatic bladder cancer and helps people with cancer.

When I called her shortly after my diagnosis, she was a compassionate listener and told me all about her experience with having an internal artificial bladder. She is also very active on the Bladder Cancer Café list-serve. I wish her continued wellness.

10 EPILOG

My experience with bladder cancer between 1997 and 2010 has been documented fully on my website and in my book, *Stop Cancer in its Tracks: Your Path to Mindfulness in Healing Yourself³*. This book is available as a PDF by request.

I think it is worthwhile for you to read a summary of that first episode along with a summary of the 2013 episode. You may choose to skip this chapter if you wish.

ONSET OF DISEASE

On Super Bowl Sunday in 1997, I showed up with a serious muscle invasive bladder cancer. Before I even knew what it was, I began to do research on the internet and learn about what serious blood in the urine meant. By the time I received my diagnosis, I could point my doctor to a document I had printed with the precise diagnosis.

I immediately began looking for integrative medical practices that could increase my chances of surviving the cancer. The *gold standard* for muscle invasive bladder cancer is to perform a radical cystectomy, an operation that removes the bladder, prostate, and lymph nodes. I opted for "The Road Not Taken" and decided on a bladder-sparing protocol involving transurethral resection of the bladder tumor (surgery), radiation and chemotherapy.

I consulted with Michael Broffman at the Pine Street Clinic (innovators in dogs sniffing cancer) and Dr. Martin Rossman, MD of the Collaborative Medical Center about the wisdom of such an approach. Michael advised me that even if the bladder-sparing protocol did not work, I could still fall back on the radical cystectomy. He also recommended Chinese herbs and supplements that were timed precisely to the stages of treatment that I received from the medical profession.

Throughout the recovery period of this first episode, I participated in many forms of integrative medicine, all substantiated by my daily meditation practices. I had guided imagery sessions, acupuncture, massages, faith healers, Reiki and much more.

I took part in many support groups such as one with the world famous dancer, 94-year-old Anna Halprin (see *Reach Out to Others*). Perhaps you have heard of the marvelous work she has been doing in the world. As I write this, she is preparing to go to Israel to foster peace between the opposing parties.

Another memorable support group was at the Center for Attitudinal Healing, founded by Dr. Gerald Jampolsky.

RETREAT WITH THICH NHAT HANH

In August, 1997, I went on retreat with Zen Master Thich Nhat Hanh at the University of California, Santa Barbara. I spent about 30 minutes talking with Sister Chan Khong in the dormitory courtyard about cancer and I told her the little poem that came to me in an extraordinary guided imagery session. The session took place on the spring equinox.

Two days later, I was walking down to the beach with Thay and the sangha. I watched Thay as he sat on the dune and mindfully drank his tea. Something in the way he sat moved me to hold his hand on the way back to the dining tent. This felt like a massive dose of healing for me and I am truly grateful for this opportunity.

By the middle of 1998, I was in remission, but that was not the end of all cancer. In 2000, I traveled to India on business and stopped in Plum Village (where Thay resides) on the way back.

FIRST RETURN OF CANCER

When I returned to California, I learned that there was carcinoma in situ in my bladder. This was treated with very little difficulty using a tuberculosis vaccine known as BCG instilled directly in the bladder. After six treatments, the cancer was once again gone.

On September 13, 2001, Thay gave a lecture in Berkeley. We were all disturbed by the events of 9/11, but Thay's lecture brought us a moment of peace. The next Sunday, we had a Day of Mindfulness at the Spirit Rock Meditation Center near my home. I remember the feeling of tears in my eyes as Sister Chan Khong led us in *Touching the Earth*.

GIVING BACK TO MY COMMUNITY

Then on the summer solstice of 2009, I founded the **Mindfulness in Healing**[1] sangha, which has been meeting every week since then. My sangha sister and OI member, Carolyn DeFay or I have been there every Wednesday night except when it falls on a holiday. Today, Mindfulness in Healing is a thriving, wonderful sangha with a small group of committed members and consistent leadership.

MORE CANCER EPISODES

This brings me to 2010. In the spring of that year, I, once again, had carcinoma in situ in my bladder. This minor episode was also treated successfully with BCG.

But in December of 2013, I had no such luck. Several transurethral surgeries and biopsies revealed that I once again had muscle invasive bladder cancer.

Dr. Neuwirth sent me immediately to the University of California in San Francisco Medical Center to perhaps the number one urologic oncologist in the USA, Dr. Maxwell Meng, MD. His advice: remove the bladder, i. e. perform a radical cystectomy.

I had to find a better way.

I opted for neoadjuvant chemotherapy; that is chemotherapy prior to surgery, to buy some time. I had no idea that the chemotherapy would be so toxic. I only had half of the recommended number of doses and I found recovery to be very difficult.

It was at a visit with Dr. Meng that he stopped the chemotherapy and wanted to proceed to the radical cystectomy within four to eight weeks. I was still weak from the chemotherapy and continued to explore alternatives.

To the team of Michael Broffman and Dr. Martin Rossman, I added Dr. Roger Morrison, MD – a homeopath, and Dr. Sara Gordon – a doctor of oriental medicine. Michael Broffman recommended and provided the Chinese herbs and supplements I take. Dr. Rossman treated me with acupuncture and served and my primary care physician. Dr. Morrison provided me with a revolutionary homeopathic remedy based on research by Dr. Ramakrishnan in India. Dr. Gordon provided me with additional supplements containing turmeric and spent many hours with me in meditation in our monthly Shabbat sangha and in our home.

With a team like this, I set out to once again eliminate muscle invasive bladder cancer. Dr. Meng was obliging and offered me the alternative of surveillance. This involved a cystoscopy – a scope that is inserted in the bladder to look for lesions and other indications of cancer. When he said, "I don't see anything I would want to remove," I was happy but knew this was not the end of this episode.

The cytology report revealed carcinoma in situ once again and he recommended BCG. This was administered by Dr. Neuwirth, my doctor in Marin and completed at the end of August.

On Monday, October 13, 2014, I had the follow-up cystoscopy and got the results two days later: The cytology was benign. I had once again gotten rid of muscle invasive bladder cancer with all my body parts intact.

SEVEN PRINCIPLES OF MINDFULNESS IN HEALING

I have written *Healing with the Seven Principles of Mindfulness: How to Thrive and Succeed in a Complex Cancer System* in order to inspire people with all kinds of diseases to become their own advocate for health care. I feel that it is important for people to participate in their healing experience and not just roll over and let the medical establishment run over them.

I believe that anyone diagnosed with a serious illness should investigate alternatives, as I have done and choose the ones that they feel will work for them.

I know that it is important for people to make lifestyle changes to accommodate their new life situation. This may include abstaining from sugar, gluten, meat, dairy, and other SAD (Standard American diet) food substances. This may also include mindful movements and other forms of exercise like Tai Chi and Qi Gong.

I urge them to take on a daily mindfulness practice so that they can withdraw themselves into themselves and become aware of what is really going on in their bodies, feelings, sensations, and mind. I recommend that they follow my blog, **Meditation Practices**.

I have often recommended that people gather their family and friends to help support them through difficult times. This includes joining support group like a sangha or one specifically oriented to what ails them.

I have found that having a team of medical practitioners who know both Eastern and Western methods indispensable for my own healing. They have pointed me in the right direction over the past 18 years.

I propose that when people are ready, they should try to give back to the community that supported them during their recovery period. This will give them the same sense of joy I experience in leading the **Mindfulness in Healing** sangha.

These, in a nutshell, are the seven principles of mindfulness in healing.

Will you please join me in helping people understand how they can utilize these principles for the healing experience and their life?

CLOSING REMARKS

In the Buddhist tradition, we have a practice of sharing the merit of whatever we do. In this case, I offer the following verses:

May the merit of our practice, suffering and recovery benefit all beings and bring peace.

May you be safe from internal and external harm.
May you have a calm, clear mind and a peaceful, loving heart.
May you be physically strong, healthy, and vital.
*May you experience love, joy, wonder, and wisdom in this life, **just as it is**.*
May all beings be happy, truly happy.

11 ABOUT THE AUTHOR

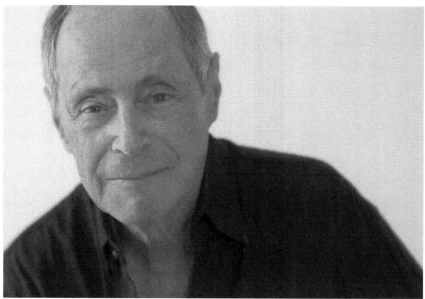

Dr. Jerome Freedman is an author, healthcare advocate, mindfulness meditation teacher, and a cancer survivor since 1997. He is a long-time practitioner in the tradition of Zen Master Thich Nhat Hanh in which he is an ordained member of the Order of Interbeing. His recent article in The Mindfulness Bell titled "Healthy and Free" touched many people. He is also a certified teacher of the Enneagram in the Oral Tradition with Helen Palmer.

Jerome currently teaches **Mindfulness in Healing** at the Pine Street Clinic in San Anselmo, California and writes daily on his blog, **Meditation Practices**. He is a contributing author of *I Am With You: Love Letters to Cancer Patients*, Nancy Novak, PhD, and Barbara K. Richardson.

Dr. Freedman served on Board of Directors of the Marin AIDS Project and the Advisory Council of the Institute for Health and Healing between 2007 and 2010. He is now a major contributor to the Buddhist Climate Action Network and the Plum Village Climate Response as an activist promoting earth protection.

Dr. Freedman holds a Ph. D. in computer science, along with two master's degrees in physics and a bachelor's degree in chemical engineering. He still consults internationally on software engineering problems and expert witness cases. He successfully interviewed Dr. Neil deGrasse Tyson on cosmology and Buddhist thought in 2011.

He can be reached by for consultations, dharma talks, lectures, and days of mindfulness by email at jerome [at] mountainsangha [dot] org.

ALSO BY DR. FREEDMAN

Stop Cancer in its Tracks: Your Path to Mindfulness in Healing Yourself

Seven Steps to Stop Interruptions in Meditation: How to Concentrate and Focus on Your Meditation and Deal with Distractions

Cosmology and Buddhist Thought: A Conversation with Dr. Neil deGrasse Tyson

The Enneagram: Know Your Type! Awaken Your Potential!

Contributing author to *I Am With You: Love Letters to Cancer Patients*[19] published February, 2015.

GUIDED MEDITATION RECORDINGS

Anger Control Guided Meditation

Achieve Goals Guided Meditation

Sound Sleep Guided Meditation

Stress Relief Guided Meditation

Reduce Symptoms Guided Meditation

Weight Loss Guided Meditation

Order from mountainsangha.org/products.

12 DEDICATION

This book is dedicated to my family –

  Mala, my wife of more than 32 years

  My son Micah

  My daughters Rachael and Jessica

  To Zen Master Thich Nhat Hanh

  And

  To all the many practitioners who helped me along the path to recovery.

13 ACKNOWLEDGEMENTS

First and foremost I want to thank my family for their continued support throughout my healing experience.

My wife, Mala, was always there for me – through pain and sorrow, happiness and joy. She went to every appointment and held my hand during the chemotherapy infusions. She brought me food and drink when I couldn't get out of bed. She helped me limp around after the surgery on my thigh and shoulder. I don't know what I would have done without her.

Then I want to thank my children, Micah, Rachael, and Jessica. The children were always around and they did not seem to be too worried. In June, 1997, Rachael graduated from Marin Horizon School to go on to high school. I remember how much I cried during the speech she gave during the graduation ceremony.

Thanks also go to my sister, Brenda Pyka, and brothers Manuel, David, and Joe Freedman for their love, support, and thoughtful visits.

I am ultimately grateful to Zen Master Thich Nhat Hanh for providing me with the inspiration and insights that allowed me to pursue my path to well-being with an attitude of taking life just as it is and meeting adversity with equanimity. Big thanks also go to the brothers and sisters in the Order of Interbeing as well as the current and previous members of the **Mindfulness in Healing** sangha. Special thanks go out to Chan Phap Vu for his generous permission to use his photograph as the cover background image.

In addition to Thich Nhat Hanh, I want to thank Phillip Moffitt for giving me Buddhist teachings from a different perspective.

Also, I want to express my gratitude to Nancy Novak, PhD and Barbara K. Richardson, editors of *I Am With You: Love Letters to Cancer Patients* and the editors of the *Mindfulness Bell* for allowing me to tell a bit of my story in their publications.

Then I must thank my healers.

Dr. Martin Rossman was a true friend and splendid healer for me. He attended the meeting when Dr. Neuwirth pronounced my diagnosis and treated me throughout 2014. I am totally grateful to him for his support and thoughtful foreword.

Michael Broffman served as my guide and quarterback through conventional and alternative treatments. I am really grateful for all he has done to help save my bladder and recover from cancer. I am also grateful for his generosity in allowing or weekly sangha gatherings to take place at the Pine Street Clinic since 2009.

Dr. Sara Huang, MD was actually the person who may have had the most significant impact on saving my bladder. She is a longtime family friend and head radiation oncologist St. Mary's Hospital in San Francisco. Sara connected me with Dr. William U. Shipley, MD, whose bladder sparing protocol played a pivotal role in my treatment.

Leslie Davenport provided psychological support for Mala and me during the whole ordeal. Her work with me with interactive guided imagery and other techniques allowed me to find some inner resources to facilitate resilience and insight. You read about the guided imagery session on the spring equinox of 1997.

Anna Halprin played a wonderful role in my healing experience. Her movement and art support group was truly something I'll remember for the rest of my life. Long live Anna, now 95 and still teaching!

The Center for Attitudinal Healing, founded by Dr. Gerald Jampolsky, provided healing support for both Mala and me. The sessions there were very worthwhile.

My team of doctors, Dr. Harry Neuwirth (urologist), Dr. David Gullion (oncologist), Dr. Francine Halberg (radiation oncologist), Dr. Robert Belknap (family doctor) were all wonderfully supportive and helpful during my crisis months. To my surprise, they all cooperated in administering the Shipley bladder sparing protocol and I am eternally grateful for their efforts.

Dr. Maxwell Meng and Dr. Charles Ryan, in addition to Dr. Rossman, Dr. Roger Morrison, Dr. Sara Gordon, Michael Broffman, Dr. Neuwirth, and Dr. Gullion, were members of my team for the most recent episode. Dr. Meng was the quarterback of the standard medical treatments and Michael Broffman for the alternative medicine. I am totally grateful for all of their efforts.

There are many other people that deserve a huge round of applause for their contributions to my well-being. Specifically, I want to mention Kushi and Linda Kullar, Dr. Israel Rios, MD, Carolyn de Fay, Gary Gach, Lyn Fine, Lorna Saas, Anila Manning, Douglas Childers, Dr. Sara Gordon, DOM, Maryanne and David

Raynal, Jessica Zerr, Simone de Winter, Julie and David Bernard, Clare and Dana Ullman, Judy Dominici, Janice and Larry Carson, Ramona Mays, Goldie Curry, Anita Morse and Dr. Steve Morse, PhD, and Dr. Geoffrey Saft, DC for attending meetings with doctors, visiting me, participating in the healing circle and meditation sessions, advising me on this book, and many other helpful activities. Most, if not all, are mentioned in the above pages. Please do not underestimate their importance in my healing experience.

A special acknowledgment goes out to Dr. Patricia Frisch, PhD for helping me see the value of using "complex" in the subtitle.

I am also indebted to the people who gave generously to the Indiegogo campaign to help cancer patients and their caregivers cope with their diagnosis by receiving free copies of *Healing with the Seven Principles of Mindfulness* and the many people who have signed up to receive these free copies.

Last, but not least, I want to thank the people who wrote reviews included in chapter 14, "What People are Saying." They are Dr. Kelly Turner, PhD (author of *Radical RemissionI)*, Julie Bernard, Dana Ullman, Alicia Dunams, and Henry Dahut. These reviews helped complete the design of the cover.

Thank you one and all and may you experience love, joy, wonder and wisdom in this life, just as it is.

14 WHAT PEOPLE ARE SAYING

"Dr. Freedman speaks from experience, both as a cancer survivor himself, and the father of a Radical Remission cancer survivor. His book, "Healing with 7 Principles of Mindfulness" gives readers a nurturing, helping hand throughout the entire cancer journey, especially with regard to developing a meditation practice."
-**Kelly Turner**, PhD, Author of the NYTimes Bestseller "Radical Remission: Surviving Cancer Against All Odds"

I am a 19 year parotid gland cancer survivor, a type of cancer that can return at any time. In addition to traditional western medicine protocol, as part of my healing process, I have used many different alternative healing modalities. The approach that Jerome has documented in his book coincide with my experience of surviving cancer. His book is a great resource for anyone facing the trauma and challenges of a serious health crisis.
--Julie Bernard, Homeopath

"Jerome Freeman's "Healing with the Seven Principles of Mindfulness" is a user-friendly approach to make practical (very practical!) specific things that can empower each person to achieve higher levels of health. These principles are not just logical and rational, they work...and they just feel 'right.' These principles will not only improve your health, they will improve your life!"
--**Dana Ullman**, MPH, CCH Author of 10 books, including two that contain a Foreword by the Physician to Her Majesty Queen Elizabeth II, "The Homeopathic Revolution," "Discovering Homeopathy," and "Everybody's Guide to Homeopathic Medicines" (co-authored with Stephen Cummings, MD)

I have reviewed your Indiegoogo campaign[20] page and book. Miracle! Truly, the story of your son will touch the hearts of millions.
Your vision of the book being available to those diagnosed with Cancer is admirable, and something that I greatly align myself with. As someone who recently started meditating, I see the healing effects of mediation, and would love to share it with the world.

--**Alicia Dunams** Author of Goal Digger: Lessons Learned from the Rich Men I Dated

This book is great! Dr.Freedman allows the reader to journey with him as he harnesses the power of mindfulness to heal himself from Cancer. He also brings the reader along with him as he carefully and meticulously considers the many options of both alternative and traditional healing approaches. The Seven Steps is both "practical" and "spiritual". Especially the part of having your friends and loved ones being an essential part of your healing journey. Would recommend this book to people going through health challenges, as well as r those who want to obtain a greater insight into the power of mindfulness.

--**Henry Dahut, J.D**. Author of Henrys Puzzle - Awakening To Infinity.

15 REFERENCES

Dr. Martin Rossman, M. D.
Medical Doctor, Author of *The Worry Solution* and other books, Acupuncture, Guided Imagery
1341 S Eliseo Dr
Greenbrae, CA 94904
thehealingmind.org

Michael Broffman, L. Ac.
Expertise in Eastern and Western cancer treatments
Acupuncture, Chinese Herbs, Supplements
124 Pine Street
San Anselmo, CA 94960
pinestreetclinic.org

Dr. Roger Morrison, M. D.
Medical Doctor, Homeopathy
80 Nicholl Ave
Richmond, CA 94801
herrickmorrison.com

Dr. Sara Kendall Gordon, L. Ac., DAOM
Functional Medicine, Acupuncture, Meditation
sarakendallgordon.com

Dr. Sarah Huang, M. D.
Radiation Oncology, St. Mary's Medical Center, San Francisco
stmarysmedicalcenter.org

Dr. Geoffrey Saft, D. C.
Chiropractic, Hyperbaric Oxygen Therapy
hyperbaricoxygenca.com

Dr. Sarita Shrestha, MD, OB/GYN
Ayurveda
saritashrestha.org

Jessica Zerr
Yoga Teacher & Massage Practitioner
backtotheessencebody@gmail.com

Simone de Winter, MA, Certified Ayurvedic Specialist
CYT, CMT
911R Irwin Street
San Rafael, CA 94901
www.marinayurveda.com

Leslie Davenport
Guided Imagery, Institute for Health and Healing
1350 South Eliseo Drive, Ste 120
Greenbrae, CA 94904

Dr. David Gullion, M. D.
Medical Oncologist
1350 S Eliseo Dr
Greenbrae, CA 94904

Dr. Francine Halberg, M. D.
Radiation Oncologist
1350 S Eliseo Dr
Greenbrae, CA 94904

Dr. Maxwell Meng, M. D.
Chief of Urologic Oncology, UCSF
1600 Divisadero St.
San Francisco, CA 94115

Dr. Harry Neuwirth, M. D.
Urology
1000 South Eliseo Drive
Suite 201
Greenbrae, CA 94904

END NOTES

[1] **Mindfulness in Healing** sangha (meditation group) takes place on Wednesday nights from 7:00 – 8:30 at the Pine Street Clinic, 124 Pine Street, San Anselmo, CA 94960. All are welcome.
    For more information, see www.mindfulnessinhealing.org.
[2] "Mind Stories Helped Cure Cancer", **Meditation Practices**: www.mountainsangha.org/mind-stories-helped-cure-cancer/
[3] *Stop Cancer in its Tracks: Your Path to Mindfulness in Healing Yourself,* Jerome Freedman, PhD, 1997, 2014. For more information, visit www.mountainsangha.org/stop-cancer-in-its-tracks/
[4] **Meditation Practices for Healing and Well-Being** can be found on the web at www.mountainsangha.org.
[5] *Cancer – The Forbidden Therapies* is a documentary film. You can read about it and watch it at www.mountainsangha.org/suppressed-cancer-cures/
[6] *The Search for the Cures Continues...* is a series of eleven documentary films produced by The Truth About Cancer and Ty Bollinger. Write me if you have difficulty locating the list of 28 practitioners interviewed in the series.
[7] *Strengthening Your Immune System Through Mind and Movement* by Shirley Dockstader, MA, Marghe Mills, MED, and Dr. Richard Shames, MD. Order from the Pine Street Clinic website: www.pinestreetclinic.com/strengthening-your-immune-system-through-mind-and-movement/
[8] *Mindful Movements,* created by Zen Master Thich Nhat Hanh
[9] Hoffman Institute, hoffmaninstitute.org, a 6 ½ day psychospiritual retreat delving into obstacles from your past. Highly recommended.
[10] *Anticancer: A New Way of Life,* David Servan-Schreiber, M.D., Ph.D., Viking, 2009.
[11] *Hungry for Change,* A Documentary Film About Creating Lasting Weight Loss, Abundant Energy and Vibrant Health
[12] *Origins,* a documentary film about helping people understand the intrinsic connection between their lifestyle, their health and the vitality of our planet.
[13] "First Mindfulness Meditation Practice", www.mountainsangha.org/first-mindfulness-meditation-practice/.

[14] **9 Minute Meditation**, the path to well-being is on the web at www.2wellbeing.org

[15] These verses were from a video on YouTube featuring Jack Kornfield.

[16] *Love is Letting Go of Fear*, by Dr. Gerald G. Jampolsky, MD, Crown Publishing Group (Random House), 1979, 2004, 2011

[17] *Emotional Intelligence: 10th Anniversary Edition; Why It Can Matter More Than IQ*, by Daniel Goleman, Bantam Dell, 1995-2006. See, for example, www.mountainsangha.org/daniel-goleman-on-emotional-intelligence/ and his other book, *Social Intelligence: The New Science of Human Relationships*, by Daniel Goleman, Bantam Dell, 2006.

[18] *Mind Over Medicine: Scientific Proof that You Can Heal Yourself*, Lissa Rankin, MD, Hay House, 2013, p. 60, **bold faced** phrases are mine for emphasis.

[19] *I Am With You: Love Letters to Cancer Patients*, edited by Nancy Novak, PhD and Barbara K. Richardson

[20] Indiegogo campaign: igg.me/at/7

12759744R00083

Printed in Poland
by Amazon Fulfillment
Poland Sp. z o.o., Wrocław